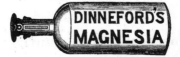

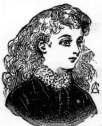

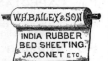

Children Thrive on Bovril.

Bovril is a "safe" food; even the tenderest baby can be given it with advantage. It is ideal for building up the little frame, for giving firm bone and muscle.

"13, Thrope Road, Staines, Middlesex.

"I am quite sure that BOVRIL was the means of saving my baby's life last year. When he could take nothing else, he never refused BOVRIL, and he has had it daily ever since. I am pleased to state that he is as well and strong as anyone could wish for.

"Believe me, yours faithfully,

(Signed) "M. LEVETT."

Icilma.

Icilma Natural Water, Icilma Soap, and Icilma Fluor Cream are a perfect boon in the nursery. When used on babies with and after their bath they prevent catching cold, and strengthen the skin against irritations, chilblains, etc. A constant use of Icilma Fluor Cream will give a lovely skin, sweetly perfumed with a delicious flower scent.

A few drops of Icilma Water cure immediately cuts, burns, insect stings, and prevent the swelling and discolouration of bruises. Icilma Natural Water is harmless, and approved by the highest medical authorities. It contains exactly the delicate combination, so difficult and costly to obtain by art, of natural salts (*vide* "Lancet" Bulletin of the Paris School of Medicine, etc.) required to make a perfect skin tonic.

PRICES:—

Water, 1/-, 2/-. Soap from 5d. Fluor Cream from 1/-.

ICILMA, 142, Gray's Inn Road, LONDON, W.C.

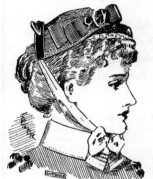
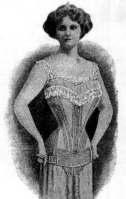

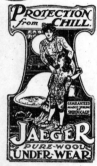
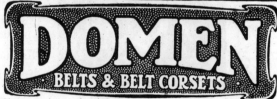
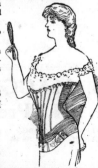

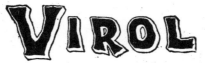

First Published 1891
Copyright © in this edition 2007
Tempus Publishing Limited

Tempus Publishing Limited
The Mill, Brimscombe Port, Stroud, Gloucestershire, GL5 2QG
www.nonsuch-publishing.com

British Library Cataloguing in Publication Data.
A catalogue record for this book is available from the British Library.

IISBN 978 0 7524 4234 1

Typesetting and origination by Nonsuch Publishing Limited
Printed in Great Britain by Oaklands Book Services Limited

OUR BABY:

FOR MOTHERS AND NURSES.

BY

MRS. J. LANGTON HEWER,

CERTIF. OBSTETRICAL SOCIETY, LONDON ; LATE HOSPITAL WARD SISTER.

NINTH EDITION, REVISED.
FORTIETH THOUSAND.

BRISTOL : JOHN WRIGHT & CO.
LONDON : SIMPKIN, MARSHALL, HAMILTON, KENT & CO., LIMITED.

1904.

Introduction

Every expectant mother wants to know the best way to bring up and look after her child. It is as true today as it was a century ago. Nowadays, we have almost unlimited means of finding out information – from books, magazines, the internet and television – but in Edwardian times the choice of where to find out information was limited. In 1891, even before Dr Benjamin Spock was born, and a good half a century before his seminal book on child rearing, Mrs Langton Hewer wrote *Our Baby for Mothers and Nurses*. Chock full of information on how to bring up a baby, with chapters on what to feed and how, what to wear, childhood diseases and baby's troubles, *Our Baby* has many tips that would prove invaluable even today.

However, the book was written for the Victorian and Edwardian mother and there have been many advances in childcare since then. As a result, we shouldn't automatically take its contents as gospel. Some chapters will amuse, some will contain valuable advice, while others would be considered downright strange today. Make your own mind up but enjoy reading how the Victorian and Edwardian mother coped with their own little bundles of joy.

PREFACE TO THE NINTH EDITION.

THE present, or Ninth Edition, of ten thousand copies of "Our Baby" is the largest yet printed. Such a steady increase in the demand is gratifying proof that the little book still finds friends, and fulfils the purpose for which it was written.

The whole has been thoroughly revised and re-set in new form for this issue; and a few head lines and leading words have been added in prominent type to facilitate rapid reference.

ANNIE M. HEWER.

Highbury New Park, London,
July, 1904.

INTRODUCTION.

IT is a fact, curious though true, that a human being may often be put to shame by the brute creation.

The mere animal seems instinctively to know how to care for and provide for its young, from the first moment of its arrival till the time that it is enabled to look after itself.

The intelligent and highly cultivated female of the human race seems, however, to be deficient in instinct on this matter. What lamentable ignorance is often displayed by a young and inexperienced mother in the bringing up of her offspring! There may be plenty of love and affection, but no knowledge.

A young mother is usually influenced a great deal by her monthly nurse, and, where the nurse is intelligent and properly trained, this is a good thing. Unfortunately, many so-called nurses have no right to the name at all; they have inherited, or invented, certain ideas on the bringing up of a baby, to which they cling with all the tenacity of obstinate ignorance.

This little book has been written for those mothers and nurses who know that there must be a right way of bringing up a child, and who are anxious to know what that right way is.

No two babies are exactly alike, and every child has its own peculiarities ; but if mothers only knew some of the general principles which underlie the successful rearing of healthy children, they would be able to alter and adapt them to each individual case. Thus, instead of being at the mercy of everybody's opinion and advice, the mother will be enabled to go on in her own way, knowing that it is the right way, and, at the same time, will have a good, sound reason for all that she does for baby, be it with regard to clothing, food, ventilation, or anything else.

It may seem a Utopian idea, but it would certainly raise the standard of health in the next generation, if every girl were obliged, before leaving school, to pass an examination on the very important subject of " How to bring up a Baby."

The medical chapters have been specially written for the book, and the whole has had the advantage of being revised by a London physician.

ANNIE M. HEWER.

Highbury New Park, London,
January, 1891.

CONTENTS.

CHAPTER VI.

BABY'S EXERCISE AND SLEEP.

CHAPTER VII.

HOW BIG OUGHT BABY TO BE ?

CHAPTER VIII.

WHERE SHALL I PUT BABY ?

CHAPTER IX.

BABY'S NURSE.

CHAPTER X.

BABY'S TROUBLES.

CHAPTER XI.

Baby's Accidents.

CHAPTER XII.

Baby's Illnesses.

CHAPTER XIII.

Medicines for Baby.

OUR BABY.

CHAPTER I.

MY BABY.

The Newborn Infant—Washing—Bathing—Dressing—Hard
Water—Care of the Skin—The Hair—Baby's Basket—Warmth
and Quiet.

A BABY, for the first few days of its life, is, as a rule,
beautiful only to its mother. Its rosy hue makes it
resemble a boiled lobster, to the masculine mind at least,
whilst its utter lack of intelligence makes it even more
uninteresting than a puppy. But to its mother, the little
tiny red morsel of humanity is already both beautiful
and precious.

If healthy it will be plump and, after washing, will
have a bloom likened to that on a ripe peach. Should it
be immature, it will be extra small, have no hair, the
nails will be imperfectly formed, and the child will
easily get chilled. If yellow and wrinkled it is probably
diseased.

EARLY WASHING AND DRESSING.

The Washing of a young infant requires great care and
gentleness. The skin is extremely delicate, and hard
rubbing, or on the other hand imperfect drying, will
chafe it. The gentle handling of a naked, newborn
infant gives it feelings of discomfort, and rough, awkward
handling even actual pain, so that all unnecessary
movements should be avoided. And as Baby becomes
very easily chilled, all draughts must be guarded against,
and lengthy ablutions eschewed.

Washing should be conducted before a fire, with a

screen round nurse's chair, and the door and windows carefully shut. Before the first bath the child should be gently smeared all over with some sweet oil, which will help to remove the greasy material with which the skin is coated. The nurse should wear a large flannel apron, while an indiarubber one beneath acts as a guard to her dress. Everything likely to be required should be placed in baby's basket within reach. The bath should be small, and be about half full of water at a temperature of 100°. It is important that the temperature be always verified by a thermometer, failing which, the nurse's elbow should be the test.

The child should be placed on its back, across nurse's knee, and be covered with a warm piece of flannel, which is not to be removed until the eyes and face have been carefully washed. The eyes must be thoroughly sponged, and the lids opened and examined to see that there is no secretion pent up behind them. The mouth should also be cleansed morning and evening with a piece of soft linen wrapped round the finger.

The whole body is then rapidly washed with a piece of flannel and plenty of soap. The child is then placed in the water, its back resting on the nurse's arm and hand. The water should cover the child entirely, with the exception of its head, and, if it enjoy it, two or three minutes may be spent in the bath. The head should of course be sponged by the disengaged hand. The child must then be lifted out on to nurse's lap, laid upon its back on a warm towel, and covered by a second. These should be very soft, and two of baby's diapers will answer admirably.

The Drying consists more in careful " dabbing " than in rubbing. After the front of the child has been dried, a little dusting powder should be rubbed on gently by the hand, especially in the folds of the groins, elbows, knees, etc., the wet under-towel being now removed, the child should next be turned gently over on its stomach, and the same process repeated.

Dressing.—As soon as the drying is accomplished the clothes must be put on, commencing whilst the child is still on its stomach, by placing on its back, first the vest, then the binder, the diaper, pilch, and flannel petticoat. The child is then turned over and the cord dressed, by dusting it with some oxide of zinc or boracic powder, and inserting it between a slit made in a small piece of antiseptic gauze, which is then folded up and the sides doubled over to form a little pad. The binder is now brought round, over the pad, and stitched together ; it is not necessary to bind the child round and round like a mummy. The diaper is then applied by bringing up its point between the child's legs, and pinning it together. It is well, however, before fastening up the diaper to grease the child in these regions. The point of the pilch is not brought up between the legs, and only its sides are pinned together. The flannel petticoat, which generally overlaps, is then tacked together, over the child's chest, the lower end being doubled back about three inches below the feet and secured by safety pins. The little frock is then pulled gently up over the feet, the arms put in the sleeves and the child turned over for the last time to have it fastened behind, and the head flannel applied.

Should this process have been carefully gone through, the child should be warm and comfortable, and quite ready to go into its warmed cradle for a long nap. A small indiarubber hot-water bottle is almost a necessity in any but the hottest weather, and should be placed in the cot, at the side of the child, between the folds of the upper blankets.

GENERAL WASHING AND DRESSING.

For the first week the child should only be bathed once a day, and that in the morning, as it is well until the cord separates to keep it and its dressing as dry as possible. The clothes should, however, be changed, and the lower parts sponged in the evening. After a week, a bath may be given with advantage night and morning, and the temperature of the morning one may be gradually lowered until in the summer, at six months old, it may be 80°. A child should love the water, and be allowed to play by splashing about and having the water sponged over its head and face.

When about a year old, if there be a large bath in the house, the child may be put into it, and after the first day or two, will probably enjoy it thoroughly. It is well, just before taking a child of this age, or rather older, out of the water, and whilst standing in it, to give a rapid sponge down with quite cold water : it strengthens him and makes him less susceptible to cold, but, until he is four or five years old it is not, as a rule, a good plan to give a perfectly cold bath. If after babyhood a bath once a day is all that can be managed, it should be a warm cleansing one at night, temperature 100°, ending with a cold sponge down, and a good rubbing with a fairly rough towel. In the morning the child should be rubbed down with a wet sponge or towel. Habits of bodily cleanliness are easily learnt, and if all young England were brought up in them from the cradle, this country would soon be considerably cleaner and healthier.

Hard Water.—If the water used for cleansing purposes is very hard it is difficult to prevent a child's skin becoming rough. In towns where rain water is often unobtainable, much of the hardness can be removed by prolonged boiling, or by the use of Maignen's anticalcaire, but even then without great care in attending to all the creases, so numerous in a fat baby, chafing will occur. Sometimes it is well to employ grease, instead of the powder, for a day or two ; if however, in spite of all care, a child gets very sore and chafed, there is probably some internal derangement, and a doctor should be consulted.

The clear soft skin is one of the greatest attractions of childhood, and, if roughened by cold winds or hard water, a little cold cream or Vinolia should be applied.

The Hair.—It is well not to wash the hair more than twice a week after baby is six months old, and then to use soft water and a little Vinolia, or other super-fatted soap.

If the skin of the head gets dry and scurfy, a little vaseline applied at night and washed off in the morning will generally cure it. After birth the hair tends to get of a lighter hue until about two years of age, after which it gradually becomes somewhat darker again. The colour of an infant's hair at birth will usually be a fair sample of what it will be in adult life. The hair will grow better afterwards if kept short for the first three years.

Water should not be allowed to enter a baby's ears, and any moisture noticed after the bath should be removed by the insertion of a scrap of absorbent cotton-wool, which without any pressure will dry the ear perfectly. It is a bad plan to try and clean the interior of a child's ear with soap and water, or with the screwed-up corner of a towel or handkerchief. These efforts only tend to push the secretion further in, until it at length presses against the delicate ear-drum, which is most undesirable.

BABY'S BASKET.

The article known as "baby's basket" is a great convenience. It should be large, stand high, and have one or more shelves beneath. It is well to have it made of brown wicker, as it keeps clean, and it is usually lined to match the cradle. A serviceable material is a pretty washing cretonne or print. It should have· a pin-cushion at either end, and several little pockets in the sides, to hold the smaller articles that are required. The basket should be completely stocked a week or so before baby is expected, in order that all may be ready when wanted. Baby's basket should contain a complete suit of clothes—as will be described—flannel apron, and six soft diapers.

The fittings proper should consist of :—

Packet of antiseptic cord dressings and powder
Packet of absorbent cotton-wool (2 oz.)
Packet of linen squares for washing the mouth
Linen thread
Needles, cotton, thimble, and blunt-pointed scissors
Turkey sponge and square of flannel in sponge bag or box
Vinolia or oatmeal soap in celluloid case
Powder box containing zinc and starch powder in equal parts, or Woolley's sanitary rose powder
Pot of grease, *e.g.*, zinc ointment and vaseline, equal parts
Large and small nickel safety pins
Allenbury thermometer, for taking the temperature of bath, food or room.*

---

* The above fittings can be obtained, packed in a box, from Messrs. Bailey & Son, 38, Oxford Street, W., if application is made for "Our Baby's Basket Fittings."

WARMTH AND QUIET.

Two important points of baby management during its first weeks of life are warmth and quiet. It must be remembered that baby has, till its birth, been accustomed to a temperature of 100°, and though 60° to 65° F. is not too low for the air it is to breathe, only the face and hands should be exposed, as, at this temperature, it will rapidly lose its bodily heat and become chilled. This will affect the general nutrition, and, in spite of food, baby will not gain in weight. Baby should therefore be kept from changes of temperature, and not be carried about the house for a fortnight. After this time it can be gradually "hardened off," though much care is required in winter (see page 67).

Quietness is also of great importance, and should be maintained for some time. A baby's brain needs to be kept from all unnecessary impressions, sudden noises, etc., and it should therefore be but little talked to. This may sound harsh, but it is a necessary warning to young mothers. An excited babyhood leads to many serious nervous diseases in childhood, and it is a good plan for at least three months. to keep the little one away from a nursery full of brothers and sisters, all anxious to nurse and play with baby.

Chapter II.

WHAT SHALL I DRESS BABY IN?

Baby's Outfit—Utility and Ornament— Anatomical — and Physiological Facts—Position of the Lungs—The Brain— The Bowels—The Feet—The Skin—Material for Clothing— The Layette—Long Clothes—Short Clothes—Walking Clothes.

THE question at the head of this chapter is not one which is left to be settled when baby has appeared. All a young mother's female acquaintances have had something to say upon this weighty matter, and a first baby generally finds an ample wardrobe awaiting it. But curiously enough, this wardrobe is only meant to last the child for three or four months, and what is to be put on at the end of that time no one has troubled to think.

Now, in the months before a first baby is born, the mother often has many quiet days and hours; and did she but know how in a year or two she would look back with longing upon those same quiet hours, she would employ them with a little more forethought. " Learning by experience " is a thing that most newly-married people get pretty well versed in after a time: but perhaps it may not be necessary, in this way at least, for some of the readers of this little book.

Baby's outfit for the first two years of life shall now be considered, and wise mothers will probably prepare some at least of the second stage garments.

What mother, rich or poor, does not like to see her baby dressed prettily? Do not some mothers, however, fail to see that true beauty cannot exist without fitness? Nature always teaches this. Animals belonging to cold countries have long, woolly, fur coats, whilst those belonging to hot countries have fine, thin, short-haired coats ; both beautiful because both perfectly fitting or

suitable. So should it be with clothing, and especially
with children's clothing.   " Trees is ornament, what we
wants is utility " was the answer of an old man in
Punch when asked why he was cutting down some
beautiful old trees.   There is some truth in the latter
part of the sentence, whatever we may think of the
former.

In the preparation of baby's wardrobe we will think
first of utility, then of ornament.

DANGERS CONNECTED WITH CLOTHING.

Many a mother has lost her child through want of a
little anatomical and physiological knowledge.   Let us
look at a few points.

(1). *The Lungs.*—Most mothers are fully alive to the
necessity of protecting a child's lungs, but how many
know that the lungs extend above the collar bone on each
side, and come down under the armpits ? Did they
know it, surely no child of theirs would go about a
draughty house, much less the draughty streets, with
such low dresses and short sleeves that both these
important parts of the lungs are exposed to the risk of
a chill, to be followed perhaps by severe bronchitis and
death.

(2). *The Skull.*—Every mother is alarmed, and rightly
so, if her child falls on its head, for fear the brain should
be injured ; but how many are aware how thin the bony
covering of the brain is ? Did they know, surely they
would not send their child out to play in the scorching
sun, or to ride in a perambulator with a hat which is
pushed far back on its head, leaving all the front part
fully exposed.   The brain, as a consequence, may become
so irritated that congestion and fits ensue.

There is preserved in one of our museums a specimen
of a baby's skull through which a cock has pecked a
hole, showing how thin must be the bone.

(3). *The Bowels.*—Many mothers are troubled by a
constant diarrhœa or constipation occurring in their
babies, who otherwise seem quite well.   The cause seems
a complete mystery, which is, however, easily solved,
when it is remembered that a child's bowels are so

delicate that the slightest chill may affect their healthy action, and that for this reason they require to be most carefully protected. Half a dozen petticoats with short waists will do no good, for if a child lie on its back and kick, the bowels will often have no protection at all. A knitted belt to reach from the hips to the armpits, and to which the diaper can be pinned, will cling to the child's body and avert all risks.

In older children a large expanse of thigh and leg left uncovered will lead to the same disturbances, and flannel drawers, fitting closely just above the knees, will give the necessary protection.

(4). *Tight Clothing.*—Chinese mothers are often condemned for such cruel bandaging of their children's feet as to stop their growth. Nearer home too, in Italy, the babies are firmly bound round and round with yards of material from head to foot, the arms being fixed to the sides, and are then placed on a pillow to be carried about like a parcel. When the time comes for them to walk, they cannot, as their legs are too thin and weak to support them, and even when they manage, after a time, to toddle along, their legs become crooked and bent.

English mothers are wiser than this, but even they do not always realize the mischief of tight clothing. Some babies are compelled to vomit their food, on account of their tight inelastic binders, which prevent the expansion of the stomach ; whilst others cannot take a deep breath nor yawn without pain for the same reason. Some children too, can only walk a few yards because of the weight of their boots, or on account of their little toes being cramped up in an unnatural position.

(5). *The Skin.*—Everyone has heard of the naughty boy who painted his dog all over, the poor creature dying in a few hours. But how many mothers have thought how important an organ the skin must be if the cessation of its functions cause death.

Many a child is unable to perspire properly and get rid of its extra heat, from the weight of non-porous clothing which has been heaped upon it, while many another has caught a chill from the contact of its skin with cold substances, *e.g.*, linen, or cotton, soaked through with perspiration.

WHAT CLOTHING SHOULD BE.

These five points will have shown a thoughtful mother that the nature of a baby's wardrobe must not be left to mere chance to decide. It must be chosen and made up on clear definite principles, principles indeed which involve the little one's health and comfort.

Thus, all important internal organs must be carefully protected from external changes of temperature.

Large surfaces of skin must be covered, as a superficial chill often causes internal disorders, and the greater the loss of heat from the exposure of large surfaces, the more will require to be generated internally to make up the loss, so that the food which ought to be making the little one fat and plump, is diverted into the production of heat to keep it alive.

All clothing should be porous and light, to allow the skin to act freely ; and should, at the same time, be somewhat elastic, fitting the part closely but not tightly.

The material selected should be one that will retain the body heat to some considerable extent, especially remembering that the younger the child, the quicker it loses its natural heat. Without doubt the substance that best adapts itself to these requirements is *wool*, and the well-known Dr. Jaeger's system is based on this theory. The very mention of the word " wool " dispels the idea of muslins and laces, which seems naturally to connect itself with a baby's outfit.

The Jaeger Company sells a baby's outfit, or " layette " as it is called, composed throughout of wool, or one can be made at home.

SCHEME OF CLOTHING.

A simple scheme of clothing for the first two years of life will now be given, based upon correct principles, and while it will form a sound foundation, each individual mother can improve upon it as she will.

The outline shall come first, and a few explanations be given afterwards.

(*A*).—LONG CLOTHES—32 Inches.

 4 Vests of fine woven wool
 2 or 3 Flannel Binders and 2 Woven Belts
 4 Flannel Petticoats or Long Flannels
 4 Woollen Night-dresses
 4 Silk or Woollen Dresses
 6 Flannel Squares or Pilches
24 or 36 Turkish Towelling Diapers
 3 Head Flannels
 1 Shetland or Knitted Shawl
 1 Woollen Hood
 4 Pairs of Knitted Shoes
 1 Veil

(*B*).—FIRST SHORT CLOTHES—23 Inches.

Larger Vests of fine wool, knitted or woven, but with long sleeves and high necks, thicker in winter than in summer
Larger Belts, knitted or woven
 2 Pairs of Flannel Stays
 4 Woollen Petticoats with bodices
 4 Night-dresses
 4 Silk or Woollen Dresses
 4 Pairs of Woollen Socks with long legs
24 Larger Diapers
 6 Pairs of Flannel or Knitted Drawers
 8 Bibs

(*C*).—FIRST WALKING CLOTHES—21 Inches.

 3 Pairs of Combinations
 4 Woven Belts
 2 Pairs Flannel Stays for winter, or
 2 Pairs Flannel Straps for summer
 6 Pairs Knickerbockers
 4 Woollen Petticoats
 4 Frocks

The first list will look very meagre when compared with the ordinary layettes advertised, but one advantage of a woollen outfit is that the garments do not crease so quickly, and they are also best washed at home. If the rule be followed that all clothing worn be first aired by an open window and afterward by a brisk fire before being again put on, the flannel garments will not need washing so often as those of linen or cotton; and one vest, petticoat, dress and nightdress will thus often last a week.

(A).—LONG CLOTHES.

Vests.—The best are soft woollen ones, being less irritating than the hand knitted. They can be obtained at all good outfitters, with long sleeves and opening a short distance down the front, but some especially suitable for young infants, opening the whole way down the front, can now be made to order. It has been amply demonstrated that muslin shirts are unnecessary even at first.

Binders and Belts.—A strip of flannel, 5 by 18 inches, is used at first, but woven belts which need no stitching are recommended after a fortnight. They can be obtained at any of Jaeger's, or the Greenock knitting depots. Good knitters can easily make them, as they resemble knee-caps.

Long Flannels.—These should be of soft, fine flannel —six yards making four petticoats. Pryce Jones, Newtown, N. Wales, keeps a good flannel called the Eureka, which, in the finest quality, washes and wears well. The bodices should have shaped shoulder straps which button and prevent the petticoat slipping down, or else be made with shoulder seams. Long flannels are generally embroidered all round.

Night-dresses.—These should serve also as monthly gowns and be daintily made. The material can vary with the season. For a winter baby, Eureka flannel is the best ; for a summer one, gauze flannel from Pryce Jones, or a good nuns' veiling. The latter can be obtained at the stores or the larger drapers, and being of double width is very economical.

Dresses or Robes.—These, if care be bestowed on them, can be made as pretty as any mother can wish, and will be far more cosy and soft than starched muslin.

Gauze flannel, llama, a material resembling *mousseline de laine,* to be obtained at the Army and Navy Stores, good nuns' veiling, fine cashmere, and washing silk, can all be utilized. Smocked fronts and wrists are always becoming to infants, or embroidered yokes and wristbands, with tucks and embroidery on the skirt, and soft torchon lace as a trimming. A sash of the same material can be added if liked. *Silk* as a material for outer garments can be recommended, as it retains heat much better than cotton, and has no starch to irritate the skin.

Flannel Pilches.—Welsh flannel is considered to be the best for these, which are about 27 inches square, and have button-holed edges.

Diapers.—Woollen diapers are advised by some, but provided they are frequently changed, fine cotton or Turkish towelling ones answer just as well and are less liable to irritate the skin. The latter need not be ironed, and are easily washed.

Head Flannels.—It is well to provide at least one of large size. Pryce Jones has a flannel 45 inches wide for this purpose, also one of 36 ins. wide for the smaller ones.

Shawl.—A large white Shetland shawl is a delightful article, possessing the maximum of warmth with the minimum of weight, and when soiled can be cleaned to equal a new one, but it has the drawback of being expensive. A fine crocheted or knitted shawl is the best alternative, and answers for an outdoor wrap far better than the usual ornamental cloak hanging over the nurse's arm.

Knitted Shoes are generally presented in sufficient number by Baby's friends.

Hood.—For both boys and girls this should be woollen, a simple one being made of a long piece of single knitting with large needles and Shetland wool. This is doubled over several times and the front rolled back and secured with ribbon.

Veil.—This is required in cold or windy weather, and should be of silk or wool. The practice of laying a linen handkerchief over a child's face is most pernicious. A sunshade is needed in sunny weather.

An out-door set, in which the cloak, hood, and robe are all in one, has been devised by the Alioné Company. This can be easily slipped on over the other clothes, and saves time, as well as unnecessary movement.

(B).—FIRST SHORT CLOTHES.

These are generally needed by healthy children when ten or twelve weeks old in the summer, but not for a

few weeks later in the winter. It is better to have a
new long-clothes outfit for each new comer, with the
exception perhaps of some of the long flannels, so that
if expense be a consideration the short clothes can
mostly be evolved from the long ones. It is important
that the shortening be gradual, the clothes reaching four
inches below the feet at first ; and as Baby ought still
to be carried lying down quite flat, this length will be
found to be convenient.

Vests and Belts may not yet require renewal, as they
differ only in size.

Stays.—These are made of two layers of flannel, and
may be quilted with a machine, thin in summer, thick in
winter. The armholes are bound with flannel binding.
They should cover the collar bone and reach to the
hips.

Petticoats.—These are made with long-waisted bodices,
the skirt consisting of a frill sewn to the bodice. The
neck is high, and in very cold weather sleeves to the
elbow are required. For summer wear, cashmere, nuns'
veiling, or gauze flannel are recommended, and for
winter, twill or Eureka flannel or one of the good unshrinkable flannels such as Viyella. The lower edge can
be embroidered or trimmed with lace.

Night-dresses.—The long ones can generally still be
used, though they may need new yokes and wristbands,
but if they are made of the thinner woollen materials
which were worn over long flannels, the latter must be
retained, unless the weather be hot, when a vest beneath
will be sufficient.

Dresses.—The long frocks can have a piece cut out
above the tucks, an extra one being made to hide the
join, or, in a plain skirt, the hem can be turned up again
and half a dozen tucks be put in. Smocks will generally
have stretched sufficiently to last a few months longer,
but yokes will probably require renewal. Later on,
when old enough to keep warm by playing, there is no
necessity in summer weather for sleeves below the elbow ;
remembering, however, what has been said about the
position of the lungs, the upper arm ought always to
have a woollen covering. The coloured unshrinkable

flannels are very suitable for these dresses, as, though washing well, they require it less frequently.

Socks.—Those known as three-quarter length are best, and in winter should be worn as well as the ordinary wool boots. A little later small pieces of morocco leather or kid can be easily fashioned into dainty little shoes, and when a child can toddle leather shoes can be worn, but they must be very soft with broad and thin soles. Shoes are better than boots for little children, as the ankles are not confined, with moderately thick soles for outdoor wear, and in winter gaiters to the knee. While a child is well wrapped up in a perambulator, the fewer outdoor garments the better, to lessen the wearisome operation of dressing to go out.

Drawers.—These, whether made of flannel or hand-knitted, should be worn over the diaper, buttoned to the stays, and reaching just above the knee. They obviate the necessity of a knitted petticoat, and are far superior in warmth.

(C).—WALKING CLOTHES.

A child is generally ready for these at about two years old, some earlier, if they are forward and big for their age.

Night-dresses.—These should now give place to *pyjamas*, made all in one to button at the back. They obviate all risk of cold, the child being unable to kick them off. Viyella is a good all-the-year-round material. It should be supplemented in winter by a long woven vest, worn beneath, as children generally lie with arms and upper part of chest uncovered.

Belt.—Same as before.

Combinations.—These should be of pure wool, woven or knitted, thick in winter with high necks and long sleeves, thin in summer with high necks and short sleeves. They can be obtained with the lower part made to button up at the sides, and while reducing the number of garments required, are equally suitable for girls and boys.

Stays or Braces.—The former, which have already been described, can be replaced in very hot weather by straps of double flannel, 23 inches by 1½, stitched each side, with buttonholes at the ends, the knickerbockers having four buttons, two in the front and two behind to correspond. The straps pass over the shoulders, crossing each other back and front.

Knickerbockers.—Flannel or cashmere in winter, nuns' veiling in summer.

Petticoat.—This should be long waisted, resembling the short coating one.

Frock.—Let this be high necked, with sleeves to elbow or wrist, according to the season ; made with a yoke into which the skirt can be gathered for girls, and box-pleated for boys, is the simplest method, while smocks are always becoming.

OUTDOOR CLOTHING FOR CHILDREN.

The more exercise a child takes when able to run about, the less clothing is required to keep it warm, perspiration tending to weaken the system and render it more liable to chills. Clothed in one layer of wool from neck to knees, with the additional protection of the belt to the sensitive abdominal organs, a child of this age in very hot weather only requires additional clothing for the sake of appearance. For this reason silk or cotton upper garments are generally preferred for summer wear in towns.

For seaside or country wear, when a child runs alone, and may choose to rest upon damp grass or wet sand, only woollen clothing is admissible, and the simplest garb consists of combinations and belt, flannel stays or straps, knickerbockers and frock. The two latter should be alike, and made of woollen beige or fine serge. The frock should hang straight from a yoke, confined at the waist by a belt into which when crawling or paddling the skirt can be tucked.

At this age it is of great importance that in summer the whole head should be well protected from the sun's rays. Large pith hats with turned-down brims can be obtained, which shade well and yet provide for plenty of air beneath. A cabbage leaf in the crown is a homely but useful precaution.

Pinafores have not been mentioned, as they have no direct bearing upon health, except that overalls, in which a child can do whatever it likes, are much to be commended as aids to muscular development and healthy appetite. Made of blue serge, or red turkey twill, they are almost indestructible.

Samples and paper patterns of all the garments mentioned in this chapter can be obtained from Miss Burn, 196, Green Lanes, London.

Chapter III.

WHAT SHALL I FEED BABY ON?

Nature's Food—A Mother's Duty and Diet—Treatment of
Mother's Nipples—Regularity of Meals—Composition of
Milk—Suckling—Cracked Nipples—Excess of Milk—Why
does Baby cry?—Cramp—Colic—Hunger—Bottles—Twins—
When a Mother should not Nurse her Baby—Weaning—
Diet Tables—Beef Tea—Variety in Diet.

IT has become too much the fashion of late years for
mothers to deliberately decide not to nurse their
babies, quite forgetting that, having brought a child into
the world, it is their simple duty to give to that child the
nourishment which nature has provided.

It is wonderful to see how perfectly nature has
adapted this nourishment to the every want of a child.
For the first few weeks the mother has only the amount
of milk that so young an infant needs ; after a time she
has more, and of a stronger quality, because the child
needs it. When baby is about nine months old the
mother's milk becomes poorer in quality and less in
quantity. Why ? It is nature's sign that the child
now requires more food than the mother can supply,
and is an indication for her to wean it. This is as nature
means it to be; but, sad to say, in an age of hurry and
skurry, hard work and insanitary customs, it is very
seldom practically realized.

How many pale, thin, weary-looking mothers are met
with, all their strength exhausted in the production of
food for their infants, and this food unfortunately being
only half as nourishing as the babies require ; their
puny condition bearing sufficient testimony to their lack
of nutriment !

Such things ought not to be, and would often be
averted by a little more common sense and care, both
before and after baby's birth.

A hand-fed baby's life is threatened with numberless drawbacks and dangers, to which a breast-fed baby is not even exposed. Poor breast milk is, of course, worse than cow's milk ; but the point to be striven after by every mother who is anxious to do her duty to her child is that her milk should not be poor but good ; and she should endeavour, by every means in her power, to provide nature's own nourishment for her helpless infant.

THE NURSING MOTHER.

The average woman of the present day cannot fulfil this duty without a considerable amount of care. Even before the child's birth she must endeavour to place herself in as perfect a condition of health as possible ; not by lying in bed, but by taking daily outdoor exercise, and by continuing her household duties. She should at the same time feed up well on simple articles of food, such as milk, eggs, fish, and meat.

She should also prepare her nipples for the arduous duties so soon to fall upon them, by bathing them night and morning, for two months previous to the child's birth, with a mixture of equal parts of brandy, or spirit, and glycerine. Spirit alone makes the skin hard and liable to crack. If the mother have small and depressed nipples, it is well to pull them out regularly at the time of bathing them, and to carefully avoid any pressure upon them.

Years ago women were treated, after confinement, on the starving system ; but this has proved to be a mistake. A mother who wishes to feed her baby must feed up well from the beginning. Supposing the child to have been born during the night,—at eight o'clock the next morning the mother should be ready for a breakfast of bread and milk, or bread and butter with cocoa ; at eleven, a lunch of beef-tea and toast ; at one, a dinner of poached or boiled egg and milk pudding, or bread and butter ; at half-past three, a cup of tea with plenty of milk or cream in it ; at half-past five, a cup of cocoa and bread and butter ; and at half-past eight, a supper of beef-tea, gruel or soup. During the night, a pint or a pint and a half of milk or gruel should be taken.

This kind of diet should be continued until the third or fourth day, when the bowels will probably have been relieved, after which, fish or meat may be taken for dinner and supper, and bacon or fish added to the fare at breakfast, after the preliminary cup of bread and milk, gruel, or porridge.

All food must be easy of digestion. Cooked fruit and vegetables may be taken in moderation, but pickles, acid drinks, highly-seasoned dishes, and raw vegetables, carefully eschewed.

The question of stimulants at this time is one upon which there is a diversity of opinion. Spirits and wine should certainly never be taken, except as a medicine ; but if a woman is accustomed to beer or stout, one or even two glasses a day may prove beneficial. In a few instances stout, though not taken at any other time, may, if drunk at dinner and supper, promote the flow of milk by helping digestion. On the whole, great dislike to malt liquor is a sufficient reason for not having it, and in such instances, if persevered with, it has generally been found to disagree with baby. In these cases two, three, or even four pints of boiled milk either given alone, flavoured, or made thick with corn flour, barley, oatmeal, or rice, will do far more good both to mother and child.

If a mother means to nurse her child she must count the cost. Hot places of amusement, irregular or late hours, must be resolutely abandoned, and she will be unable to leave home for more than two or three hours at a stretch unless she takes baby with her. Regularity in feeding is one of the great secrets in the successful rearing of infants, and must never be interfered with by pleasure.

The nursing mother should also avoid any excitement and worry. The character of the milk is often much altered by mental disturbances, and, in extreme cases, it has caused convulsions. Should a mother be much upset from any unavoidable cause, it would be well for her to draw off the milk with a breast-pump before again allowing the child to take the breast. A bottle of boiled milk and water will do the child less harm than the disturbed milk of the mother.

After the first month, gentle out-door exercise may be taken, but as the mother's internal organs do not return to their normal condition for about eight weeks, no violent exercise should be indulged in before that time. Some hours of each day should, however, be spent lying in the open air, or before a widely opened window, well wrapped up.

The good milk of its mother, then, is the best food for every infant, because it is nature's provision, suited for every want.

Human milk consists of certain substances, in certain proportions which are necessary for the growth of a child. These proportions will vary slightly according to the richness or poverty of the milk, but a fair sample would give as follows :—

Water	..	..	..	887	parts
Nitrogenous elements, *i.e.,* casein				23	,,
Milk sugar	..	..	..	63	,,
Fat	..	..	..	24	,,
Salts	..	..	..	3	,,
				1,000	,,

'These elements are in the exact proportions required to nourish a baby, and at the same time exist in such a state as to be easily digested by the infant. The first day or two after baby is born there is no proper food secreted, but a thin watery fluid which is called colostrum. This fluid has the purgative action which is required by the child, and which is quite sufficient for its needs, no butter and sugar, or castor oil, being called for.

If very hungry a few teaspoonfuls of sweetened milk and water may be given until the milk comes, but usually it is not needed.

NURSING BABY.

A mother should nurse her child every five or six hours until her supply of milk comes, and afterwards every two hours *by the clock*, from 6 A.M. to 10 P.M.

After 10 P.M. it is well from the very beginning to accustom a child, unless exceptionally delicate, to go as long as possible without food ; four hours is the usual time, thus it will come to its mother at 2 A.M. and again at 6 A.M. Some children are more easily taught this rule than others, but perseverance will always win the day. Infants' stomachs need rest, and night is the time for it.

On the second or third day the mother will probably be hot and restless, and will feel her breasts enlarge with the incoming milk. She should at once begin to feed the child regularly every two hours, giving each breast alternately, one side being sufficient for a meal.

Whilst nursing baby the mother should not sit up in bed, as that may cause faintness, but should have a second pillow to raise her a little, and turn slightly towards the side from which the child is going to suck. The infant's head should rest upon her arm, and she must put the first and second fingers of the opposite hand above and below the nipple, to prevent baby's little nose being so pressed upon that it cannot breathe.

A vigorous baby sometimes nearly chokes itself in its haste, and it may be necessary to occasionally withdraw the nipple for a moment to allow it to get breath. A weakly child, on the other hand, may not suck strongly enough, but steady firm pressure on the gland may cause a quicker flow of milk, and so assist the infant. Ten or fifteen minutes usually suffices for a meal, at the end of which time the child will generally fall asleep with milk escaping from its lips. It should at once be removed from the mother and placed upon its right side in the cradle. The right side is chosen, as the distended stomach will not then press upon the heart. It is of the greatest importance that the child's mouth should be then closed, and thus the good habit of breathing through the nose be early established.

After each nursing the nipple should be gently sponged with warm water, thoroughly dried, and then painted with the brandy and glycerine mixture. The slightest crack on the nipple should at once be treated, as, if neglected, it may lead to an abscess of the breast, and such intolerable suffering that nursing has to be abandoned. It is advisable, for a day or two, if any cracks have appeared, to use a glass or indiarubber nipple shield, enlarging the hole at the end of the teat that the child may get the milk easily. If there is great difficulty in making the child suck with a shield, the milk can be drawn off and given with a bottle. The crack itself should be kept thoroughly dry, be frequently painted with Friar's balsam or tannic acid in glycerine, and touched occasionally with a piece of blue stone, all applications being washed off before nursing.

For the first few weeks the flow of milk is about a pint in the twenty-four hours; in later months it may reach three or even more pints. Some mothers, especially at first, have more milk than the child can take, and it runs away, causing great discomfort. In such cases it is well to increase the solid but diminish the liquid food, and to press the surplus milk out of the breast before the child takes it, as the milk which has been the latest secreted will be the best. It may even be well to draw off some of the milk with a breast pump, if it be giving rise to fever, bad headache, or mental disturbance, but things usually right themselves in a day or two, and the demand will equal the supply.

A weakly baby will, as a rule, take less milk at a time than a strong one, and, in such a case, one and a half hour's interval in the day and three hours' at night may be required for a week or so; but, as soon as possible, it should be put on the ordinary hours.

After the first month two-and-a-half hour intervals are not too long between each meal during the day, retaining the four or five hour interval during the night. A healthy child will sometimes sleep six hours at a stretch during the night, to the great advantage of both parents and offspring.

WHY BABY CRIES.

Some mothers complain that baby is "always crying," and they therefore conclude it is always hungry; but, in point of fact, there are many reasons why a healthy baby may cry, and it may be well to consider a few of them. Baby may cry, because :—

(1). It may have been too long in one position and is cramped.

(2) It may have a tight band somewhere, or a pin, with an unprotected point, running into it.

(3). It may be too hot or too cold.

(4). It may have the wind or the " gripes."

(5). It may be hungry.

Now before supposing the last to be the case, unless indeed baby's food is really due, it is best to exclude the other four reasons.

The proper remedies will be :—

(1). Turn baby over on its other side in the cot and turn its pillow.

(2). Examine its binder, also examine the safety pins and see that they are quite secure, of course assuming that no one is allowed upon any pretext to put ordinary pins into the child's garments.

(3). Feel if it be hot and perspiring; if so take off a blanket or head flannel ; if on the other hand, it be chilly, take it up, warm it by the fire, wrap it in a hot blanket, and put a hot-water bottle in its bed, before laying it down again.

(4). Place the child over your shoulder, gently rubbing its back, or put it upon its stomach on your knee ; if it bring up the wind freely it will be comforted, and probably drop off to sleep.

If this be insufficient, and the child's face be of a bluish hue, its eyes and mouth twitching, and its extremities cold, while its cry is peevish and in paroxysms, give it half a teaspoonful of dill-water in two teaspoonfuls of hot water, and the attack will probably soon be over. Should baby have brought up any sour smelling milk or curds, delay the next meal, even if due, for at least half an hour, so as to give the digestion a rest ; of course, if the mother has been persuaded to give baby " just a little," it will probably stop crying for a short time, simply because the warm fluid proves grateful, but very soon matters will be worse than ever. Why ? Because the mother has been adding fuel to the flames ; baby's digestion is at fault, and, instead of giving the stomach a rest she has given it still more work to do.

(5). The child will probably have just awoke from a sound sleep, and its cry will be loud and continuous, whilst it will take the breast eagerly and steadily.

If a child awake crying frequently, *e.g.*, every hour, and yet has no symptoms of wind or sickness, and takes to the breast eagerly, the milk is probably poor in quality, even though it may be sufficient in quantity. The mother should, in such cases, try to improve the quality of her milk by taking more nourishing food, *e.g.*, eggs, cream, milk, meat, etc., and, at the same time, a tonic, *e.g.*, Kepler's Extract of Malt, may be beneficial if the appetite be poor.

The weekly weighing day must be considered the best criterion as to whether the milk be nourishing the child properly. If, week after week, there be no increase in weight, even though the child seem contented, a doctor should be consulted, who will probably examine some of the milk and decide if nursing should be given up.

A baby will sometimes take its food very well, but immediately afterwards will scream, draw up its legs, have a good deal of wind, and afterwards green diarrhœa. Here there is something wrong with the milk ; perhaps the mother has eaten some indigestible food, or drunk something acid, or may need an aperient. Any such cause must be removed, but, if the same effect be continually noted, and the child does not gain in weight, it is probably one of those rare cases in which the mother's milk does not agree with the child, and it must be weaned or have a wet nurse.

INSUFFICIENT MILK.

It frequently happens that after the mother begins to resume her ordinary duties and get about a little, the supply of milk falls off in quantity, and the child cannot get sufficient to satisfy it from one breast. The quality is excellent, but the quantity is insufficient. The child will suck until it is tired, then doze off, and, at the first attempt to move it, will wake again and suck furiously ; and then drop the nipple with rage at not being able to get what it wants. In this case the mother should arrange her food so as always to have had some nourishment about half-an-hour before baby wants a meal. A glass of rich milk, some gruel, cocoa, or beef tea may all assist.

If, in spite of all that can be done, the supply runs short, baby must have two or three bottles daily of diluted cow's milk, as will be explained later on.

It is a popular delusion that cow's and mother's milk do not agree. The mistake has arisen from the cow's milk not having been properly given. Let baby have every sixth or third meal from a bottle as is necessary, but let it be given regularly and systematically, or the child will suffer ; thus, right breast, left breast, bottle, and so on. It must be remembered that every ounce of good mother's milk is a clear gain to the child.

On the other hand, a baby should have one bottle daily after three or four weeks, even though the mother have plenty of milk ; otherwise, should the mother be unavoidably called away for a few hours, or have the misfortune to suddenly lose her milk, there will be great difficulties—a baby being a most conservative little person.

The nursing of a baby by its mother has, so far, only been considered from the baby's side of the question, and once again one would reiterate that it is of the utmost importance, at any rate for the first few weeks, that the little one should have that perfect nourishment which nature has provided for its use.

Sometimes, however, instead of one baby to be fed, there are two, and rare indeed must it be to find a town woman in the nineteenth century who is robust enough to feed twins successfully. In such an event it is well to divide the breast milk between them, and give bottles alternately with the breast ; if the one twin be more puny and weak than the other, it may be well to bring up the stronger of the two wholly by hand ; but frequently the poor mother's horror at such a rapid increase in her family causes what milk there is to disappear, which unfortunately settles the question.

There are some conditions under which a mother should not nurse her child :—

(1). If she be consumptive or markedly scrofulous.

(2). If she be suffering from any acute disease, *e.g.*, typhoid fever, inflammation of the lungs.

(3). If she be in a state of great general debility.

(4). If, after a fair trial, she have excessive back-ache, faintness, continued prostration ; or if her periods should return at all profusely.

WEANING.

The process known as weaning, in a baby who, though breast-fed, has taken one bottle at mid-day since a month old, will give no trouble. This bottle should at first consist of one ounce of milk and two ounces of barley water, the milk being gradually increased in quantity until at nine months it may be taken pure. At six months a teaspoonful of Mellins', or Savory and Moore's food should be added to this bottle ; at seven months the food can be increased to a dessert-spoonful. and at nine months weaning should begin in real earnest. Should the mother's milk be of an exception- ally satisfying nature and produced at little or no detriment to her own health, weaning may be postponed for another couple of months. Some mothers go on nursing their children till they are fourteen, sixteen, or eighteen months old, but this is a grave mistake ; bad for the child and still worse for the mother.

Supposing that the weaning is begun at the ninth month, it should be effected by adding a morning bottle to the mid-day one, a week later by giving an evening one also, and then by quickly increasing the number of bottles, until, by the beginning of the tenth month, the bottle has been entirely substituted for the breast. At this age, supposing the child sleep all night and will take nine or ten ounces of milk at a time, six bottles will be ample, as that will give nearly three pints of milk ; but this is the maximum quantity, and a small child will probably only take two and a half pints. A diet list will be given suitable for the eleventh and twelfth months.

If a child have not been accustomed to a daily bottle from an early age, weaning is apt to be a troublesome process. Should it be urgently required, it is best to do it abruptly, or endless will be the battles, and it will be best for the mother to entirely hand over the feeding of the child to someone else for a few days. Hunger will soon bring the child to the bottle; the food in this case must not be given too strong at first, but mixed according to the table for a month or so younger, and then gradually increased. Should there be no special urgency, however, and the child be very obstinate about the bottle, it will be best to gradually teach it to drink out of a cup at once, and not try it with the bottle at all. Of course it must be remembered that feeding by a cup is a much slower process than by a bottle, and unless the nurse or mother be very persevering, the child will not get its proper allowance of milk, and if it have much less than three pints at this age it will not get on.

DIET AT ELEVEN MONTHS.

7 A.M.	Milk, 10 ounces.
	Savory and Moore's food, a small dessert-spoonful.
10 A.M.	Ditto.
1 P.M.	A lightly boiled egg with stale bread crumbs, and a cup of boiled milk to drink.
	Alternating with half a pint of beef tea or some gravy from a joint with stale bread crumbs; or a custard made with one egg to half a pint of milk.
4 P.M.	Same as at 7 A.M.
7 P.M.	Ditto.
10 P.M.	—Ditto.

The above diet will give two and a half pints of milk without the portion at dinner. The food can be prepared twice in twenty-four hours as is most convenient, and each time must be placed in a perfectly clean jug, the morning and evening jugs being kept quite distinct and washed out thoroughly each time.

Savory & Moore's food has been mentioned as an example, but there are others which may be recommended at this age, *e.g.*, Allen & Hanburys' malted food, Neave's food, Nutroa food, Frame food, and Chapman's entire wheaten flour. Should the child have a delicate digestion, Benger's food will be the best to begin with. Directions for making the various foods will be found on the tins. Good cream added to the dietary is of great value.

Beef-tea for young children is generally made as follows : Cut up in small pieces, free from fat, half a pound of beef-steak, add one pint of cold water, and a little salt, put it into a jar or jug, cover the top with brown paper, and stand it in a saucepan of cold water on the fire, allowing the water in the saucepan to simmer for two hours. Turn it into a basin and, when cold, skim off any fat that may rise. If necessary a little sugar can be added before it is given. A still better method, which can be adopted in the nursery, is to cut up four ounces of best rump steak into strips and finely shred them. Soak for fifteen minutes in five ounces of cold water with a little salt, then heat very slowly, stirring all the time till the thermometer registers 130°. The juice will be all extracted and the meat left white. Strain and remove the fat by drawing tissue paper across the top. The albumin of beef-tea coagulates at 150°, so it should never reach this heat.

At this age bovril may sometimes replace home-made beef-tea with advantage, inasmuch as it contains certain of the nutritive properties of beef that are excluded from the latter. The special brand of " Invalid bovril " will be most readily taken, as it is devoid of seasoning.

DIET, FROM TWELVE TO EIGHTEEN MONTHS.

7 A.M.	Milk, 10 ounces. Savory & Moore's food, a small dessert-spoonful, or a rusk well beaten up.
10 A.M.	Milk, 10 ounces, with stale bread broken in, or a lightly boiled or poached egg, with stale bread crumbs and 8 ounces of boiled milk.
1 P.M.	Beef-tea or bovril with stale bread, and a saucer of custard pudding, or gravy and potato, which has been through a sieve, with a saucer of pudding.
4.30 P.M.	Same as at 7 A.M., with a Mellin's or milk biscuit.
7 P.M.	Ditto.
10 P.M.	Ditto.

DIET, EIGHTEEN MONTHS TO TWO YEARS.

	On waking (if early) Milk Food, 6 ounces.
8 A.M.	Breakfast ; Milk, 10 ounces.
	Lightly boiled egg and thin bread and butter.

11 A.M.	Milk food, 6 ounces.
	Plain biscuit, or crust of stale bread, with half a stick of best chocolate.
1.30 P.M.	Dinner; beef-tea or gravy, 10 ounces, with stale bread crumbs or toast.
	Plate of milk pudding.
4.30 P.M.	Tea; milk food, 10 ounces.
	Biscuits; or bread and butter.
7 P.M.	Supper; plate of milk pudding or cup of bread and milk.

As an alternative there may be given :—

> Breakfast; 2 tablespoonfuls of well-boiled oatmeal or wheaten porridge, rizine, semolina, hominy, etc., with 10 ounces of boiled milk.
>
> Dinner; half an ounce of underdone fresh butcher's meat well pounded up, or some white fish, or chicken, also potato or cauliflower well mashed, and plenty of gravy. Baked or stewed apple and cream.

It will be seen that the staple article of a child's diet, viz., *milk*, is still to be given in large quantities ; nothing can ever take its place for growing children of every age, and many children from a year old fail in strength and size simply from having left off their bottles, and not taking their equivalent in milk out of a cup.

Variety is to be aimed at in children's diet, but should not be carried to excess, thus : a small quantity of cocoa essence such as Cadbury's, boiled in milk, may be enjoyed, as a change, at the 4.30 meal. The pulp of a well baked apple beaten up with sugar and cream, mashed strawberries or prunes, with cream and sugar, bananas, the inside of grapes, the pips and skins being removed, or the juice of oranges, form useful and pleasant varieties after eighteen months ; but no indigestible parts of fruit, or uncooked apples, gooseberries, etc., should be allowed to young children.

Bread and Butter, except in very small quantities, should not be given before the age of eighteen months, and then the bread should be thin, with as much butter rubbed into it as possible, not simply laid on, as this last is indigestible.

A properly brought up child will not soon tire of its simple milk diet, and should it dislike the meat there is no necessity to give it, until at least two years old ; the great thing is that every child should have an abundant allowance of milk and plenty of animal fat. Should good cream be difficult to obtain, a valuable preparation is Virol, made from bone marrow—an emulsion very easily digested.

No feeding between meals should ever be allowed, either in the form of biscuits, fruit, or sweets. On the other hand, a little chocolate or barley sugar, given at bed time or directly after meals, can do no harm.

Should indigestion or feverishness occur, the child had better be restricted to its simple milk food for a day or two.

In some households it may be necessary to somewhat alter the hours, but the schemes above given may act as a guide to mothers upon which to plan their children's meals and food.

It may be mentioned that a big, forward child of sixteen months may require to be placed on the diet given for one of eighteen months ; and *vice versa*, a small child of eighteen months may, with advantage, be kept on the diet given for a twelve-months baby.

After the age of two years, when children have generally cut all their milk teeth, a special diet is not required, but for two or three years afterwards, at the least, it is wise to see that *definite quantities of milk* are taken, two pints being the minimum, and to allow no seasoned dishes, no tea or coffee, mustard, or pepper.

Chapter IV.

WHAT SHALL I FEED BABY ON NOW?

Wet Nurses—Composition of Human Milk—Composition of
Cow's Milk—Casein—Boiling the Milk—Feeding Bottles—
Necessary Apparatus for Artificial Feeding—Regularity of Feeding
—Times of Feeding—Quantity of Food Required—Raw Meat
Juice—Cream—Malted Food.

SOME poor babies are unfortunately deprived of the
food that nature intended for them. What is to be
done now? Two alternatives present themselves—a
wet nurse and a bottle.

In ninety-nine cases out of a hundred a wet nurse is
almost an impossibility, although the best substitute
for a mother's milk is certainly that of a foster mother.
But now that bottle feeding has reached such a high
state of perfection, wet nursing is a far rarer thing
than formerly. In some few cases, however, this may
be the only way of saving a child's life.

A WET NURSE.

A wet nurse should be about twenty-five years old,
and have had a child previous to the present one; her
infant should be a little older than the one she is about
to nurse, and both woman and child should be examined
by a doctor before she is admitted into the family. It
is generally possible to obtain a wet nurse from a Lying-
in hospital or workhouse infirmary, but it is a great
mistake to take a poor woman out of her usual surround-
ings and feed her up with better fare than she has had
in her life, insist on her having a pint or two of stout,
and give her nothing to do. Under this line of treatment the quality of the milk will quickly deteriorate,
and baby will suffer.

Wet nurses usually require a great deal of looking
after, and in London and big towns are often most

unsatisfactory. They are apt to be untruthful, careless, and given to drink, and upset the whole household. Of course, a wet nurse can never have a mother's feelings towards the child, and, therefore, often takes very little interest in its welfare, simply performing her duties in a routine manner for the sake of the money.

By far the best wet nurses are respectable farmers' wives, and these often really merit the name of foster mother.

BOTTLE FEEDING.

Dismissing the wet nurse, then :—How should a bottle-fed baby be managed ? and, What is to be put into the bottle ? In order that an infant may thrive, it is absolutely essential that it should have a food as nearly as possible identical with what nature provides. This artificial food must not only contain the proper elements, but they must also exist in the proper proportions.

There are three animals whose milk can be utilized for a human baby; the cow, goat, and ass; and the milk of all three contains the proper elements, though unfortunately not in the proper proportions.

Comparing them with human milk they give the following proportions :—

	Human Milk.	Ass's Milk.	Goat's Milk.	Cow's Milk.
Water - - - - -	887	903	853	875
Nitrogenous elements, *i.e.*, casein - - - -	23	17	45	43
Milk-sugar - - - -	63	64	58	44
Fat - - - - -	24	14	41	35
Salts - - - - -	3	2	3	3
	1,000	1,000	1,000	1,000

Ass's Milk.—This milk being much weaker than human milk, is not suitable for a permanent diet, but it has the great advantage of possessing a casein which closely resembles human casein in character. It is therefore easily digested, and is very useful for quite young infants if extra cream be added.

3

Welford's Surrey Dairies make a speciality of ass's milk, and will send it anywhere, but it is expensive, and must not be continued after a few months or the child will not thrive.

Goat's Milk.—This milk is very nutritious, being stronger than cow's milk in each constituent. Its casein however resembles that of cow's milk, and is equally difficult for a baby to digest. Goats are said to be proof against tuberculosis, which is an advantage, and their milk is much used abroad for infant feeding. If substituted for cow's milk in the tables given, the same proportions can be observed, but the extra cream omitted.

Cow's Milk.—This, in the vast majority of cases, is the most convenient to employ. It will be seen to contain more casein, or nitrogenous matter, and less sugar than human milk. This can easily be remedied in theory by adding water to the milk until the casein is brought down to the required amount, and then adding milk-sugar and a little cream.

Thus, cow's milk diluted with a third of water, with sugar and a little cream added, will contain not only the right constituents, but the constituents in the right proportions. At first sight all difficulties seem to have vanished, and we have made an artificial milk as good as any mother's milk. This is, however, unfortunately not the case.

WHY COW'S MILK DISAGREES.

When a child swallows its own natural milk, as soon as it reaches the stomach it is met by an acid fluid which " turns " the casein of the milk into little solid flakes. These particles are quite thin and distinct from each other, and are digested by the gastric juice, and absorbed through the walls of the stomach and intestines. When cow's milk enters the stomach, the casein, on the contrary, instead of clotting in tiny flakes, does so in large hard lumps, which the gastric juice digests with difficulty. These hard lumps or curds often pass intact through the child's intestines, setting up vomiting and diarrhœa, as well as failing to nourish it.

The important fact of the different behaviour of cow's or goat's, and mother's milk, can quite easily be demonstrated in the following manner : Place a sample of cow's or goat's milk, and another of human milk, in two glasses, and add a little acid, *e.g.*, vinegar, to both. In the glass of human milk very little change will be visible, only some tiny little flakes of casein being thrown down, whereas in the other milk large masses of curd will at once be formed.

MODIFYING COW'S MILK.

In preparing a food for infants from cow's milk it is therefore evident that we must try not only to reduce the casein in quantity, but to so alter it in quality as to prevent its liability to clot in firm masses.

Boiling the milk lessens the size of its clots, and this should always be done, not only for this reason, but because it also renders the milk less liable to undergo any fermentative changes, and destroys most of the germs of disease. But boiling the milk will not of itself render the masses of casein small enough for easy digestion, unless, indeed, the infant be blessed with extra strong powers in that way. For ordinary infants something more is required, and there are two ways in which our end may be attained.

(1). By the addition of an alkali.

(2). By the addition of a small quantity of some thickening substance to get between the particles of casein, and prevent the clotting together in such hard lumps. By the first method we act chemically on the casein, by the second mechanically. Which is the better method ?

In the first method enough alkali must be added to the milk to counteract the acid secretion of the stomach. This would require about a third of the bottle to consist of lime-water, or 3 grains of bicarbonate of soda to be added to each ounce of milk. To regularly give so much alkali as this is a bad practice, as it stops digestion for some time ; and yet to give less is of no use. The second plan, therefore, is the better, and the substances generally used are barley, oatmeal, gelatin, or one of the malted foods.

For young infants *barley* is, perhaps, the best of these mechanical aids. It is used in the following way :— Three teaspoonfuls of washed pearl barley (or one tea-spoonful of patent barley) are put into two pints of cold water, and boiled·down to a pint and a half and strained. This decoction must be used instead of pure water to dilute the milk, and must be made fresh every day, being poured into a clean jug ready for use.

Oatmeal, instead of barley, is useful where there is a tendency to constipation. Two tablespoonfuls of oat-meal should be boiled for four hours in one quart of water, and the liquid then strained through muslin, and used in the same quantities as barley-water.

If *gelatin* or *isinglass* be chosen, a piece about one inch square is put into four ounces of cold filtered water in a teacup, and allowed to stand for three hours. The cup is then placed in a saucepan half full of water, which is boiled until the gelatin is dissolved. When cold this forms a jelly, and one or two teaspoonfuls are put in each bottle.

If a *malted food* be used, Mellin's is, perhaps, the best before three months. A teaspoonful should be dissolved in hot water and added to the milk.

Again, it must be insisted upon that foods given in this way, at so early an age, are simply to act mechanically in making the casein of the milk more digestible, and not in themselves to act as a nourishment.

Healthy children of normal size, *i.e.*, weighing over seven pounds at birth and possessing fair digestive capabilities, can frequently deal with the casein of cow's milk if modified as above, especially if the mother is able to give the child a few meals a day of its own normal food. For such children the Table on next page gives the proper quantities for each meal in correct proportions.

If, however, the child be small and delicate, with no ·hope of any mother's milk to tide it over the initial difficulties of digestion, it is wisest to begin by predigesting the casein altogether before giving it to the child. This can be done in several ways, as described in the next chapter, but must only be looked upon as a temporary expedient. After about a fortnight the process must be gradually shortened, until by the end of a month the child can digest the casein of cow's milk without difficulty.

FOOD TABLE.

Age.	Meals.	Boiled Cow's Milk.	Cream.	Barley Water.	Each Meal.	Total.
3 days	10	1¼ drs.	½ dr.	6 drs.	1 oz.	10 ozs.
7 ,,	10	3 ,,	½ ,,	8½ ,,	1½ ,,	15 ,,
14 ,,	10	4 ,,	1 ,,	11 ,,	2 ,,	20 ,,
21 ,,	10	6 ,,	1 ,,	13 ,,	2½ ,,	25 ,,
28 ,,	10	8 ,,	1½ drs	14½ ,,	3 ,,	30 ,,
5 wks.	9	10½ ,,	1½ ,,	16 ,,	3½ ,,	31½ ,,
6 ,,	9	13 ,,	2 ,,	17 ,,	4 ,,	36 ,,
7 ,,	9	16 ,,	2 ,,	20 ,,	4 ,,6 drs.	42 ,,6 drs.
8 ,,	8	19 ,,	3 ,,	22 ,,	5½ ,,	44 ,,
10 ,,	8	22 ,,	3 ,,	23 ,,	6 ,,	48 ,,
3 mths.	8	3½ ozs.	3 ,,	2½ oz.	6 ,,3 drs.	51 ,,
4 ,,	8	4 ,,	3 ,,	2 ,, 5 ,,	7 ,,	56 ,,
5 ,,	7	5 ,,	3 ,,	2 ,, 5 ,,	8 ,,	56 ,,
6 ,,	7	6 ,,	3 ,,	2 ,,	8 ,,3 drs.	58 ,,5 drs.
7 ,,	7	7 ,,	3 ,,	1 ,, 5 ,,	9 ,,	63 ,,
8 ,,	7	8 ,,	3 ,,	1 ,,	9 ,,3 drs.	65 ,,5 drs.
9 ,,	6	9 or 10	3 ,,		9 or 10	54 or 60
10 ,,	6	9 or 10	3 ,,		9 or 10	54 or 60

It will be noted that cream is here added throughout the child's dietary. It has been conclusively proved that children thrive better on a higher percentage of animal fat in their food than is to be found in ordinary cow's milk. The fat must therefore be added, and its most easily digested form is cream; if this is difficult to obtain, give cod-liver oil instead, beginning with a quarter of a teaspoonful three times a day, gradually increasing. The oil must be considered as part of the child's food, and not as medicine. The lack of animal fat in infants' dietary is responsible for many cases of constipation, rickets, and malnutrition.

The percentage of fat in cream varies greatly according to the method of separating it from the milk. In large dairies the fresh cream usually contains about 50 per cent of fat. Cream which is skimmed from the top of

milk which has been allowed to stand, contains a much
lower percentage, and if this kind be used, double or
even treble the amount ordered in the Table should be
given.

With quite young infants a guarantee should be
obtained from the dairy as to the amount of fat in the
cream supplied, which should have no preservatives
added.

A small quantity of *milk-sugar* can be added to each
bottle.   It used to be considered absolutely necessary,
but if cream is regularly given it need not be insisted
upon.   All chemists supply it.

Children must be fed as to quantity more by their
weight than age ; that is, a child weighing 9½ lbs. at
birth will require more food than the Table indicates ;
but care must be taken that the same *proportions* are
observed, *e.g.*, at fourteen days 1½ times each quantity
could be measured = 6 drs. milk, 1½ drs. cream, 16½ drs.
barley water.   Here the child would have more in
quantity but the same in quality.   In the first two
months of life growth is very rapid, and the amount of
food is gradually but decidedly increased, and then more
slowly till the sixth month, when again rapid growth
begins.

If the child cannot digest cow's milk in the proportions
stated, which is often known by the passing of curds
in the motions as well as by vomiting and pain, it is due
to its difficulty in dealing with the casein, *i.e.*, the nitrogenous element in the milk.   The milk must then be
rather more diluted, but as in this case the child will
not get enough nitrogenous and fatty food each day,
these two elements must now be given in some other
way.

For the nitrogenous element *raw meat juice* is the best
thing, and, for the fatty element the cream must be
increased, or *cod-liver oil* added to the dietary.   These
are easily digested.

Raw meat juice:—To make this take two ounces of
best rump steak, obtained daily from a reliable butcher,
cut into very small pieces and place in a teacup, cover
with 1½ tablespoonfuls of cold water and stand for an

hour. Then squeeze tightly through muslin until the meat is left white and dry. Give the juice nearly cold, sweetened with a little sugar if necessary, and either by itself or mixed with the bottle. It must be made fresh, however, every day, as it quickly turns. When fresh meat cannot be obtained, Bovinine or Wyeth's meat juice is the best substitute.

The quantities of boiled milk and barley-water given in the Table (*p.* 37), will, generally, be sufficient for a child until the eighth month.

It is often advisable, especially with active, strong children, at the fourth month to give in the mid-day bottle a teaspoonful of a malted wheaten food, *e.g.*, Savory and Moore's food, and, if this agree, to add it soon to the 10 p.m. bottle also. The child will probably sleep all the better for it. At the sixth month, when growth is rapid and teeth begin to appear, the food may be added in small quantity to each bottle. It is best then to make it twice a day when boiling the milk, adding the barley water at each meal as required. Thus at six months old, when seven meals are required as per Table, the first four bottles, viz., for 7 and 10 a.m., and 1 and 4 p.m., can be prepared together, by boiling 24 ounces of milk, mixing four teaspoonfuls of Savory and Moore's food in a very little cold milk, and then pouring the boiling milk upon it, stirring it well, and returning it to the fire for a moment, but not allowing it to boil again. It must then be put into a perfectly clean jug. For each meal, six ounces of this mixture, which should not be thicker than cream, is measured into the enamelled saucepan, two ounces of barley-water is added, and it is then warmed to the required heat before being poured into the bottle.

At nine months old, instead of the mid-day bottle a cup of beef-tea or bovril may be given, with a few stale bread crumbs in it. At ten months the diet will be that of a weaned child, and has been already described.

It should be remembered that to change a child's diet because it has arrived at a certain age is not always wise. If it be regularly gaining weight, its flesh be firm, and it has a good colour, there is no indication for any change, and many infants do splendidly on milk alone until twelve months old, and on simple milk and farinaceous diet until two years old.

If any change of diet produce indigestion, as shown by vomiting, colic, or diarrhœa, it is an indication to return to the simpler food.

Regularity in feeding is one of the most important details in the successful rearing of hand-fed children. This was dwelt upon when considering breast-fed babies ; but if important with them, it is absolutely essential with bottle babies.

TIMES OF FEEDING.

An ordinary infant that is not exceptionally delicate will require feeding in accordance with the following Table.

1 Week.	1 Month.	2 Months.	5 Months.	7 Months.	9 Months.
6 a.m.	6 a.m.	6.30 a.m.	7 a.m.	7 a.m.	7 a.m
8 a.m.	8.30 a.m.	9 a.m.	10 a.m.	9 a.m.	10 a.m.
10 a.m.	11 a.m.	11.30 a.m.	1 p.m.	11.30 a.m.	1 p.m.
12 noon	1.30 p.m.	2 p.m.	4 p.m.	2 p.m.	4 p.m.
2 p.m.	3 p.m.	4.30 p.m.	7 p m.	4.30 p.m.	7 p.m.
4 p.m.	5.30 p.m.	7 p.m.	10 p.m.	7 p.m.	10 p.m.
6 p.m.	8 p.m.	10 p.m.	3 p.m.	10 p.m.	
8 p.m.	10.30 p.m.	3 a.m.			
10 p.m.	2.30 a.m.				
2 a.m.					

From the beginning, a long rest should be given to the child's stomach during the night. One bottle has, however, been allowed for in the table up to seven months, though many children will sleep from 10.30 p.m. till 6 a.m. before this. In this case the first morning bottle will require to be given rather earlier, and the other bottles a little closer together, or the requisite quantity will not be taken.

It is a good plan to always wake a healthy child, during the day, for its food, if due. After a short time it will awake punctually of its own accord. Until a child is eighteen months old it is wise to always take it up at 10 p.m. and give it some nourishment. It will then sleep later in the mornings, to the comfort of all concerned. The food should not be kept warm during the night, but heated as required, as milk readily turns if kept long at a temperature of 100°.

MILK FOR INFANTS.

The milk to be used for the hand-feeding of a baby must be chosen with care. For reasons to be afterwards given, the habitual use of sterilized milk is contra-indicated, and the dairy must be one which courts full publicity and takes every precaution against contamination.

The milk should not be from one cow but from a mixed herd, as the slightest ailment in the one cow would be far more likely to disagree with the child than if taken mixed with other milk. It should be delivered in fixed quantity morning and afternoon, in cans or bottles belonging to the customer, with the name clearly marked upon them. These cans should be sealed before they leave the dairy, and should be thoroughly cleansed with hot water and soda before being returned to the milkman. The cream must be sent in small air-tight glass bottles.

Cow's milk should be neutral, but that from stall-fed cows is often acid, and may seriously upset the child. It should therefore be periodically tested, and the easiest way is to obtain from a chemist a packet of blue litmus paper, a small piece of which dropped into any acid fluid will turn pink. If in an emergency it be necessary to use such milk, lime-water or a little bicarbonate of soda must be added until the acidity is neutralized—as can be demonstrated by the paper.

The milk should be boiled as soon as it is brought into the house. It is the only animal food which is regularly taken in England without being cooked, and, remembering the number of dangers which it may be the means of conveying, it is a necessary rule in every house (especially in large towns) in which milk is taken in any considerable quantity.

Scarlet fever, typhoid fever, diphtheria, and tubercular diseases may be contracted through drinking contaminated milk, but boiling is an effectual safeguard.

The *sterilization* of milk, instead of merely *boiling* it, has latterly much come into vogue.

Sterilized milk is milk so treated that all its germs have been destroyed, so that suitably preserved it will keep sweet for an indefinite length of time. To do this it is necessary to keep it at a certain high temperature for a lengthened period, and to seal the vessel in which it is prepared with a plug of cotton wool, which is not air-tight but germ-tight, *i.e.*, it prevents any germs in the air gaining access to the fluid.

There are various forms of apparatus on the market to enable this to be done at home, though all large dairies prepare sterilized milk to order. One apparatus consists of small bottles (each to hold a child's meal), which, kept steady in a frame, are lowered into a large saucepan of water. When required for use the cotton wool plug is taken out, and a teat slipped over the mouth of the flask. Another has an inner vessel to hold a pint or more of milk at a time, with an outer one for the water, and fitted with spirit lamp complete, but the principle is the same in all.

From careful investigations it appears clear that sterilized milk is more easily digested than simply boiled milk, which, with very delicate infants is a great advantage. On the other hand, the prolonged heating necessary has the most serious disadvantage of lessening the antiscorbutic property of milk ; therefore, children fed only upon it for some months are apt to develop scurvy, and signs of malnutrition. It thus much resembles condensed or prepared milks, and while most useful for a time in certain cases of weak digestion, is not to be recommended for prolonged use. As a matter of fact, milk which is brought rapidly to the boiling point, as usually done, has all the ordinary disease germs destroyed, while its quality is not deteriorated, and for common use is therefore perfectly satisfactory.

As soon as the milk has been boiled, it should be put into a perfectly clean jug and taken upstairs, as it should never go near meat or other contents of a larder.

APPARATUS NECESSARY.

The apparatus required for Hand Feeding is as follows :—

> A large tray
> An enamelled basin
> Two feeding bottles with extra teats and valves
> Two jugs holding 1½ pints each
> Ten-ounce measure marked in ounces
> Two-ounce measure marked in drachms
> An enamelled or aluminium saucepan
> Strainer
> Thermometer
> Blue Litmus paper
> Bicarbonate of soda tablets (3 grains each)
> One yard of muslin*

A spirit lamp or gas ring will also be necessary.

The Tray is recommended so that everything necessary will be at hand and can be moved about as required. It should stand on a table close to a widely opened window on the cool side of the house, away from drains or gullies.

The Basin is to be filled with water, and be large enough to hold the two feeding bottles, the two jugs, and little bottle of cream.

Feeding Bottles.—These should be devoid of tubes. In one of the American States it has been made illegal to use or sell bottles with tubes. The bottle should have a large teat fixed on one end, and an opening to allow the entrance of air behind the milk, such as the Allenbury bottle. Teats will often require a cross-cut to be made with the scissors, if the child suck feebly. Several of these should be used in rotation.

The Jugs—one to contain the boiled milk, the other the barley water. They should have necks large enough to allow the hand to pass in entirely for cleansing purposes.

Ten-ounce Measure.—This will be needed when the quantities exceed two ounces.

Two-ounce Measure.—This must be marked in drachms

---

* The whole apparatus, made as far as possible in white enamel, can be obtained packed in a box from Bailey & Son, 38, Oxford Street, if enquiry be made for the Hand-Feeding Outfit.

to ensure the exact quantities being given, The inaccuracy of spoon or cup measuring is responsible for many attacks of indigestion. Sufficient for one meal only should be mixed at a time. 1 drachm = 1 teaspoonful ; 4 drachms = 1 tablespoonful or half an ounce ; 8 drachms = 2 tablespoonfuls or 1 ounce ; 20 ounces = 1 pint.

An Enamelled or Aluminium Saucepan, to warm the food either by direct or indirect heat. The former is the quicker method, as the food itself is heated in the saucepan, but owing to the very thorough washing required afterwards it is not so safe as the indirect method. Here the food is measured into the bottle, which is heated by standing it in the saucepan of hot water.

Strainer.—This should be of enamel, and is necessary to prevent any of the skin of the milk passing into the bottle.

Enamelled saucepans, if used for heating by the direct method must be carefully watched, as they crack easily, and small pieces of the enamel may be detached and pass into the feeding bottle. If straining is always carried out, of course no harm would follow. Aluminium saucepans, though more expensive, are free from this danger.

Thermometer.—The one mentioned in Baby's Basket Fittings is the best. The food should register over 100° in the saucepan, as the coldness of the bottle will reduce it several degrees. The thermometer can be slipped into the neck of the bottle just before the teat is drawn on. The food should never be given to an infant colder than 99°, and it may be necessary with a very young baby to re-heat the bottle during the meal by standing it again in the saucepan of hot water.

Litmus Paper.—The use of this has been described.

Bicarbonate of Soda.—This is useful in tablets of known strength. Three grains to each ounce of milk given for a few bottles on the first sign of indigestion will often arrest an attack.

The Muslin is to throw over the tray and all its contents to prevent dust, etc., falling into the milk.

Once a day all the jugs and bottles, basin, and tray, must be thoroughly scrubbed in hot water and soda, and after each meal the bottle, teat, and whatever else was used in preparation must be well washed in hot water, and the bottle and teat replaced in the basin of cold water. Too much care can hardly be exercised to maintain the most scrupulous cleanliness in everything pertaining to baby's food, as one drop of stale milk may cause putrefaction to occur in the whole of the next meal, and frequently sets up vomiting and diarrhœa. Bottle brushes are not safe things to use ; the bristles easily become detached and may be swallowed, and cases of lead poisoning have been reported from washing out a bottle with shot.

When giving a young child the bottle, the infant must be held in a half-reclining position upon the mother's arm. From five to ten minutes must be taken over each meal, and, if the child suck quickly, the teat should be momentarily withdrawn from the mouth occasionally.

The practice of sitting a baby up and patting it vigorously on the back in the middle of its quiet meal is a bad one. It may be well, when the bottle is finished, to raise the child for a minute or two before gently placing it in its cradle on its right side, but it should always be kept very quiet after a meal.

This chapter will, it is hoped, give intelligent mothers and nurses a clear insight into the rational feeding of those little ones who are unfortunately deprived of the nourishment intended for them by nature, and if it is used as a ground plan it can be modified as occasion requires for the individual baby.

Chapter V.

WHY DOES NOT BABY GET ON?

Signs of Baby Getting On—Want of Cleanliness—Want of Air
—Want of Proper Food—Irregular Feeding—Improper Feeding
—Starch Foods—Malted Foods—Condensed Milk—Ass's Milk
—Humanized Milk—Peptonized Milk—Bread Jelly—Meat Juice
—Cream.

THE two preceding chapters describe how a healthy baby should be brought up, but there are so many poor babies in the world that do not " get on " that it may be well to go a little more into detail. How does a mother know if her baby is getting on ?

Of course, the question can at once be answered in the negative if baby is getting thin and weakly, is repeatedly having attacks of vomiting, diarrhœa, and colic, is perpetually crying and rarely sleeping ; but though none of these may be present, we cannot safely say baby is " getting on " unless most of the following signs are noticeable :—

1, A steady weekly increase in weight.
2, A firm condition of the flesh, and colour in the cheeks.
3, A good appetite at meal times.
4, Long quiet sleeps.
5, General contentment, and vigorous exercise, which it takes by kicking and stretching.
6, The teeth appearing at the right times.

The point is, *Why* does not baby " get on " ? Well, in nine cases out of ten the mischief has something to do with the diet. It may, however, be that the child is starving for want of fresh air ; there may be no ventilation in its sleeping or living room, and it may be kept too much indoors. This point has been fully dealt with elsewhere, but is again mentioned because of its importance.

Supposing, then, that baby has plenty of fresh pure

air, is well bathed in warm water every day, is warmly but lightly clad, and yet does not " get on," we must go back to the all-important question of diet.

There are, at least, four distinct reasons connected with diet why a baby may not " get on," and in only one of these can the fault be laid at the poor child's own door.

1, A want of cleanliness.
2, Irregular feeding.
3, Improper, including insufficient, feeding.
4, An unusually weak digestion.

1. The necessity for *cleanliness* has been fully treated of. But it is so very easy for a busy nurse or mother to drift into careless ways, quite forgetting that some remains of milk left in a teat or dirty jug may cause fermentation and set up vomiting and diarrhœa. In summer weather this is especially true, and a superficial washing of jugs and cans is often the reason why the milk turns so soon.

2. *Irregular feeding* is sure to be followed by evil consequences. The stomach of an infant is a very delicate organ, and quickly resents being left empty for hours at one time, and at another having two or three meals put into it in quick succession.

Baby should be fed *by the clock*, and nothing should be allowed to interfere with this rule. It is a good plan at first to write out the hours of feeding on a paper and pin it up on the wall, to serve as a reminder, but a baby fed punctually very soon serves as a clock itself.

3. But *improper feeding* is one of the commonest reasons why a baby does not " get on." Now, what are improper foods ? A very proper food for the mother may be by no means so for the infant. A little thought would soon show this. Nature provides the food on which a child ought to live for the first nine months of its life, and if this be of good quality and quantity the child thrives.

It therefore follows, as before pointed out, that a child's diet must resemble its mother's milk as closely as possible, and it may be well to consider from this standpoint some of the foods often given.

Starch Foods.—These would include pap, *i.e.*, bread scalded in water and a little milk added, arrowroot, cornflour, bread and butter, and most of the patent foods. Can any reasonable woman imagine that such things resemble mother's milk ? Yet, with many mothers these are favourite forms of diet for their babies, and then they wonder that they are such puny specimens.

The main ingredient in the above-mentioned foods is starch, a substance that infants have no power of digesting. For starch to be digested at all, even by adults, it is necessary that it should be first converted into sugar, and this is effected by the salivary glands in the mouth and others lower down. In young infants these glands are not properly developed ; and therefore while starch is a suitable food for adults, who have the power of digesting it, it is most unsuitable for infants, who have no such power, and its presence in a child's bowels only causes irritation and pain, while it affords no nourishment whatever.

Malted Foods.—In these the starch of different grains has been converted into grape sugar, which can be easily absorbed, and is valuable not only for its intrinsic nourishment, but also for its mechanical power of decreasing the size of the curd in cow's milk. Used in small quantities these foods are therefore very useful adjuncts to cow's milk, and after three months may be given freely. The same foods, however, if mixed with water only prove a starvation diet, and form a striking instance of improper feeding.

Condensed Milk.—Desiccated Milk.—Condensed milk is a favourite food with mothers, and, in very poor districts where good cow's milk is a rarity, may be recommended. The great thing necessary is to be sure the brand is one containing plenty of fat. Ignorant mothers often buy condensed skim milk, thus depriving their infants of one of the most important items in their dietary. The sweetened kinds contain a great deal of cane sugar, and babies become fat, but their flesh is soft and flabby, and their powers of resistance being weakened, any illness proves serious. The reason for this is that infants cannot take condensed milk unless freely diluted, the amount of sugar upsetting their digestion, and if much diluted both the nitrogen and fat are too lessened in quantity to properly nourish the child.

This will be seen by comparing the proportions given below :—

	Cow's Milk and Water. 1 to 1.	Condensed Milk and Water, 1 to 14.
Nitrogenous elements (casein)	21	16
Fat - - - - -	17	8
Sugar - - - - -	22	27
Salts - - - - -	3	—
Water - - - - -	937	949
	1 000	1,000

A child obliged to be brought up on condensed milk will therefore require extra *nitrogen*, in the form of raw meat juice, and *fat*, in the form of cream or cod-liver oil, to be added to its dietary, or it will be taking an " improper food," and will run the risk of rickets, delayed teething, and scurvy.

Unsweetened condensed milk can now be obtained, which is better for the child, but being less concentrated is more expensive.

Of desiccated milks one of the best is the Allenbury, prepared in two strengths, and very useful in hot weather, especially in towns, where cow's milk is apt to quickly turn. But all condensed, desiccated, and sterilized foods have the great fault of being devoid of the *fresh* element which is elsewhere shown to be a most important factor in the successful rearing of hand-fed infants.

After three months this lack can be supplied by the juice of oranges or potato gruel. The latter is made by well boiling a floury potato, passing it through a fine sieve, beating it up with milk till of the consistency of cream, and adding about a tablespoonful to several bottles a day. No mother, however, who can obtain good fresh cow's milk should rest content with condensed or desiccated milk as a permanent diet for her child.

If a voyage has to be undertaken with a baby, it is

4

well to begin with condensed or sterilized milk a few days before embarkation, that the child may have grown accustomed to the change of diet before its new trials commence.

Some babies, though their food cannot be called improper, do not have enough. These children cry out for food before the meal is due, and always seem hungry, and their napkins are seldom wet. Breast-fed babies always pass less water than hand-fed ones. More food must be given. But until a child is seven months old more than eight ounces should never be given at once.

The quality, not the quantity, may require increasing, and less water should gradually be added to each bottle until the child seems to be satisfied.

Instances have occurred of children continually craving for food : a doctor should here be called in, as there is probably something wrong.

4. The fourth possible cause is *an unusually weak digestion*. Some babies are born with very little capacity for digestion, and these, though fortunately not at all common, give a great deal of trouble to both mother and nurse.

FOODS FOR WEAK DIGESTION.

Many mothers imagine their children suffer from weak digestion, when, all the time, the fault lies not at the child's but at the mother's door : she has been treating it wrongly. It is rare for a breast-fed infant to have any great amount of indigestion ; it generally occurs in hand-fed infants, for reasons that can be easily understood from the preceding chapter.

Supposing, however, that food has been regularly given in proper quantities, and of a proper quality, and that all other reasons for a baby not thriving can be excluded, and yet the child is continually suffering from diarrhœa and vomiting, it must be concluded that the ordinary diet suitable for children with normal digestion does not agree, and that the child really has a weak digestion. Some change must be made, or it will go from bad to worse.

A good wet nurse would, of course, be the best thing to try, but this is usually quite out of the question.

Other alternatives will be :—

Ass's Milk.—This milk having a casein closely resembling that of human milk is readily digested, and is useful for a short time, but should soon have extra cream added, and it must never be continued for a permanent diet.

Humanized Milk.—In towns this is prepared at the large dairies and delivered daily, as milk is not fresh enough by the time it arrives at the consumer's house to attempt its composition at home. In the country, if cows are kept, it can be prepared by an intelligent dairymaid, as follows : Allow one pint of milk to stand six hours, take off the cream and put it into a jug, and add half the skimmed milk to the cream. Separate the curd from the remainder of the milk by means of rennet, and add the whey to the mixture in the jug, which is ready for boiling, and can be given to the child without further dilution. Should this agree, less casein must be gradually abstracted.

Mothers who have understood the preceding chapter will at once see, that though half the casein has been removed and extra fat added, yet that the casein itself is unaltered in character, and they will therefore gather that though this answers admirably with some babies, there are others to whom even the diminished quantity of casein proves an insuperable difficulty. This applies chiefly to the home-made production, the dairies partially peptonizing their mixture.

Peptonized Milk.—In fully peptonized milk all the casein and some of the fat is digested before it is taken, and the milk is thus ready for immediate absorption by the stomach. This can be effected in several ways.

1. It can be bought ready prepared from the large dairies, who send it out in bottles.

2. It can be easily prepared at home by using Fairchild's *Zymine Peptonizing Powders*, which are put up in little tubes containing sufficient to peptonize one pint of milk. Put a pint of fresh milk and 5 oz. of boiled water in a clean jug or bottle. The water may

be boiling or the milk may be slightly warm, but the temperature of the mixture must be 100° Fah. Shake into the jug the contents of one of the tubes. Put the jug into a deep saucepan or basin of hot water, temperature 110° F., and allow it to remain in a warm place from ten to fifteen minutes, at the end of which time boil it up thoroughly. The boiling stops the peptonizing or digesting process. Should the child be very ill, the process of peptonizing may be kept up for even longer than fifteen minutes, but in this case the milk will be rather bitter, and some sugar of milk must be added. It will require less dilution by one half than that given in the Table for the child's age. Peptonizing pellets, or Liquor pancreaticus, are also sometimes used to predigest the milk.

3. It can be prepared by using a preparation made by Savory & Moore, which is a condensed milk fully peptonized. This is a very convenient preparation, but it must not be used too strong, and the measuring must be done with a measure glass and not a spoon.

Either of these three methods may be followed, and if carried out carefully, will, in ninety-nine cases out of a hundred, agree with the child, the milk when entering the stomach having only to be absorbed, there being no curds of casein to digest, and therefore nothing to disagree.

On the other hand it must be remembered that though it is the right thing to feed children upon predigested food long enough to tide over a difficulty and educate the stomach, it is equally wrong to continue it for any length of time. Any organ that has no work to do, wastes or atrophies. It has been clearly shown that a healthy kitten fed entirely on predigested food, fell a good deal behind, both in weight and stature, another kitten fed on ordinary milk. Children kept too long on predigested food do not gain weight and strength as they should, and their digestive organs become weaker instead of stronger, so that it is very difficult to make any change in the diet without a violent attack of indigestion.

Peptonized food should never be left off suddenly. If methods (1) or (3) have been used, one teaspoonful of the peptonized milk should be replaced by one of boiled cow's milk in each bottle for two days, when two tea-spoonfuls can be tried, increasing by one teaspoonful every two or three days, until the whole of the peptonized milk is replaced by boiled cow's milk. If method (2) has been used, the peptonizing process must be diminished by several minutes every few days, until it can be dispensed with altogether.

CASES OF INDIGESTION.

A note of warning must be added on the subject of continually changing a young infant's food. Some mothers, who have not mastered the essential principles of successful hand-feeding, instead of seeking medical advice on such an important subject, experiment on their unfortunate baby according to the advice of the latest visitor, and are surprised that the child's stomach resents such treatment. It must not be forgotten that an acute attack of indigestion, as shown by vomiting and diarrhœa, may occur with a baby, as with an adult, from some transient cause, *e.g.*, an error in cleanliness or in the temperature of the last meal ; and the con-clusion that the whole dietary is at fault is not to be lightly arrived at. The acute attack should be treated by the *omission* of the next meal when due, to give the stomach a rest. A quarter of an hour before the second meal would be due, or earlier if the child appears really hungry, a dose of brandy according to the proportions in Chap. XIII. should be administered, and the two following bottles should consist of weak barley-water with half the white of an egg beaten up in each. This will often act like magic, by washing out the alimentary canal, and the child will be able by the time the next meal is due to take it as usual, though it is wise to make the food rather weaker than before for the next few hours. Should this simple treatment prove insufficient, it will then be necessary to try one or other of the preparations above mentioned.

Bread Jelly.—In very rare cases milk in any form may have to be discontinued for a time, and the best substitute, says Dr. Cheadle, is bread jelly. This is made by taking four ounces of stale bread and soaking it for eight hours in some cold water, then taking out the bread and squeezing all the water out, putting it into one pint of fresh water and boiling it for two hours. This prolonged boiling breaks up the starch granules and converts some of them into sugar. The pulp must next be rubbed through a fine sieve, and when cold it will form a jelly. For a meal take a tablespoonful of the jelly and mix it with eight ounces of hot water, at the same time adding a little milk sugar. Bread jelly does not keep long, and very soon turns sour.

But a child cannot thrive well if fed on bread jelly exclusively; it does not contain nearly enough of the nitrogenous or of the fatty elements. Raw meat juice may supply the one, and cream the other, *e.g.* :—

> Bread jelly mixture—four ounces.
> Raw meat juice—one ounce.
> Cream—half ounce.
> Sugar—as much as will lie on a sixpence.

The meat juice must not be added to the mixture while too hot, or its albumen will coagulate, in which state it should never be given.

The cream and meat juice may be gradually increased as the digestion improves. After a time a little boiled cow's milk should be cautiously added, *e.g.*, a teaspoonful to the bottle, and then, if no harm comes, it may be increased, so that the stomach may gradually be educated to do its duty.

All cases of very weak digestion will give a great deal of trouble at first, and though a few hints have been given, it must be remembered that infants cannot be treated by a hard and fast rule, and what may suit one might kill another. Owing to this fact, doctors now sometimes prescribe the exact amount of fat, casein, etc., which they wish the child to have, and the milk is prepared accordingly by the dairy.

The rationale of the line of treatment which will probably be adopted by the doctor will, however, be now understood, and it is an axiom that needs no proving—that unless a child have a proper amount of food, containing the proper elements, in their proper proportions, and presented to it in a form proper for its own digestion, it cannot " get on."

CHAPTER VI.

BABY'S EXERCISE AND SLEEP.

The Hardening Process—Carrying a Baby—Exercise—Crawling—
Walking—Perambulators—Going Out for a Walk—Massage—
Gymnastics—Sleep—Mid-day Nap—Hours of Sleep—Quantity of
Sleep.

EXERCISE and sleep are two very important parts of
a baby's life.

For the first fortnight very little exercise is taken,
except by an occasional stretch. After this time it
begins to be necessary for the child's health ; and that
it is enjoyed is easily demonstrated by watching a tiny
baby after its bath kicking out its legs and arms on the
nurse's knee before the fire. At this age it should be
carried in the nurse's arms for half-an-hour twice a day,
in an adjoining room in winter time, and in the garden
in summer.

The outside temperature should be at least 60° F. for
a young infant to be taken out, and if born during the
winter, it may be necessary to keep it in for some
months. If, however, the advice given on the subject
of ventilation be carried out, the child will keep quite well
and strong.

Carrying a Baby.—It should be remembered that
at birth the spine is quite straight, but will bend in any
direction that pressure be applied. The back, therefore,
must always be well supported, and, even when older,
a child should not be allowed to sit up too much, or the
spinal column, being too weak to support the weight of
the head and arms, will bend in the wrong direction.
This is one of the many reasons why it is far better for
a baby when awake to lie and kick in its cot than to be
nursed.

The " hardening process " in vogue among some mothers is certainly not good for winter babies. Until a child is eight months old it should never be sent out on misty or very windy days, especially if the wind be in the east. After this time the child may be " hardened off slowly," as the gardeners say, until it can go out regularly every day. A thick, moist atmosphere should, however, always be avoided. Children with tender skins should have a little Vinolia rubbed on their cheeks before going out in windy or frosty weather, to prevent roughness, as a clear soft skin is one of child-hood's great attractions.

EXERCISE.

Because a child cannot go out of doors it must not be left without exercise ; it should be wrapped in a shawl and taken into a room of rather lower temperature than the nursery, and carried about as before described. A tiny baby, if put on its back on a bed, will delight to kick and stretch its limbs. When old enough to run, the child should have the landing and a couple of rooms to run in and out of ; if properly clothed it will keep quite warm and enjoy the freedom.

Probably it will shout and sing at the top of its voice, giving splendid exercise to the lungs. There is some-thing wrong with a child who is always quiet ; and, at suitable times, a good noisy romp is to be encouraged.

Crawling.—Children of ten or eleven months may be put upon the floor with a few toys, and will remain happy for a long time. Little knitted overalls, combin-ing stockings and drawers, which will pull up over the feet and fasten round the waist, will admirably protect a child from cold. The draughts from beneath the door should be provided against before a child is put on the floor. Crawling seldom begins before the tenth month, and it is rendered a safe enjoyment if a Babies' Playground, invented by Mr. Abell, of Derby, is used.

Walking.—Attempts at walking are generally made at a year old, but except in thin, wiry children, fifteen months is quite young enough to begin. Should a child's legs seem inclined to bend, no walking should be allowed until a later date ; or, should bending occur after beginning to walk, the child must be resolutely kept off its feet for a time. To see a child of twenty months with bandy legs walking about everywhere, is a disgrace to its mother and nurse.

A child very easily tires ; it trots about so much in the house that its strength should be carefully husbanded out of doors. About a quarter of an hour before bringing the child in, it may be allowed to get out of the perambulator and walk or run about, but half a mile is as much as any child of two and a half years should be allowed to walk at a time. It is a great mistake to discard the perambulator too soon. It should be used until the child is at least four years of age. Over-walking is said to play an important part in bringing on infantile paralysis.

Perambulators.—How should a young baby be taken out ? This is rather a vexed question, as some people have a great prejudice against perambulators. The three-wheeled perambulators of the old style are certainly open to criticism, at least for babies under a year old, but the bassinette pattern, with careful using, is a great boon to both baby and nurse. As a matter of fact, baby is less likely to catch cold in a perambulator than if carried on nurse's arm. In the winter a hot bottle should be provided, and soft, warm wraps. The pillows should be soft, and baby be put flat on its back. In this way the child can be made as warm and cosy as in its cradle, with the addition of breathing purer air.

The child should be taken out for a walk proper, and not shopping or visiting. At first it should be kept out for an hour, and, later on, for two hours at a time. If baby goes to sleep never mind, it will not hurt it ; and, on warm summer days, it may be put in a peram-bulator in the garden, shaded carefully from the sun.

At six months old a child should go out twice a day, *e.g.*, from 11 to 1 and 2 to 3.30, in the winter ; from 9.30 to 11.30 and 3 to 5 in the summer.

Go-carts are great acquisitions to older children, they can take their turn in pushing and being pushed, and thus make their walk a source of enjoyment. To be silently pushed along in a perambulator for a couple of hours is dreary work to an intelligent child of two or two and a half. Whilst quite young, watching the trees wave about, and the carts going to and fro, was sufficient amusement, but now is the time when a bright intelligent nurse is an immense help. Children are always asking questions, and many a lesson may be unconsciously learnt while out for a walk, as to size, colour, animals, etc., by drawing the child's attention to various objects, *e.g.*, " Here is a big brown horse coming," or, " Look at that little white dog."

A large open space is a great gain to children, and should always be sought in their walks, as here the air is purer, not being contaminated by the smoke of the chimneys or the refuse of the streets. At the same time it should not be a gossip-field for the nurses, or an opportunity for their charges to mix with other children, who may come from fever-dens or vermin-filled houses.

Massage.—There is one form of exercise which little children should have frequently administered, and that is firm rubbing of the limbs upwards by the hand. This rubbing develops the muscles wonderfully, and the best time to do it is after the bath. It is specially useful in rickets.

Gymnastics hardly come into consideration when treating of babies, but a trapeze, fastened by ropes from a cross beam, is a most useful form of exercise. The Swedish exercises are of great benefit to growing children, especially girls, as their muscular development is generally but little considered, and their amusements do not naturally partake of such an athletic character as those of boys. Tiptoe exercises as soon as a child can walk, followed by skipping a little later, should be encouraged if there is any tendency to flat-foot.

SLEEP.

How much a baby should sleep is a question difficult to answer in definite terms. Generally a sleepless baby is one that is delicate, or one that has been brought up badly. When speaking of good and bad habits, it has been shown how important is the early training of an infant with regard to the question of sleep, and one can only look with pity on the nurse or mother whose bad methods of early training are bringing forth fruit in the shape of weary pacings to and fro, rocking and hushing the baby—and sometimes the " old baby " too—to sleep.

Little wonder is it that the mid-day nap is soon given up with these children ; it entails far too much labour and time.

A well-brought-up infant will for the first fortnight generally sleep the whole time unoccupied by feeding and dressing, *i.e.*, nineteen out of the twenty-four hours. At about three weeks or a month old, if encouraged to stay awake about an hour before bed-time, it will sleep better at night.

By two months old it will often be awake several times during the day for an hour at a time, but, if well trained, will be quite content to lie quietly in its cradle.

These periods of wakefulness will gradually increase until by six months a healthy child should settle off at 6.30 p.m., be taken up and fed at 10 p.m., and then sleep on till 6 or 7 a.m. ; during the morning and afternoon it should have two good sleeps of one and a half hours each, but after 4 p.m. should be kept awake to make it sleepy by bed-time.

At twelve months, a baby should sleep from 6.30 p.m. to 10 p.m., and from 10 p.m. to 7 a.m., and have a two hours' sleep in the day, from 11 to 1, or from 12 to 2.

At two years, the mid-day sleep may be shortened to one and a half hours, if the child should awake at that time, but even when it does not go to sleep, the mid-day rest should be insisted upon till five years of age. When putting the child to rest, it is best to remove its dress and shoes and darken the room.

As a general rule, little children should have twelve hours' sleep at night. It is a mistake to put a child to bed too early, unless it be convenient for it to wake at an equally early hour in the morning. Few children will sleep more than twelve hours at a stretch.

All through childhood a great deal of sleep is required, and ten hours is not too long before adult age is reached.   During sleep a child recuperates all the vast expenditure of energy which has taken place in the day ; and to curtail the former, means that the latter will weaken instead of invigorate the frame of the little toddler.

Chapter VII.

HOW BIG OUGHT BABY TO BE?

Average Weight—Average Increase in Weight—Influence of Food on Weight—How to Weigh Baby—Average Weekly Increase in Weight—Weight of Premature Infants—Average Height—Average Increase in Height—Influence of Diet on Height—Circumference of Head—Circumference of Chest—Undue Enlargement of Head.

THE weight of a new-born infant varies very considerably, the average being from about 6 to 8 lbs. The usual weight for a boy is about 7½ lbs., and that for a girl 7 lbs. A baby of 5½ lbs. would be *below*, one of 9 or 10 lbs. *above* the normal weight. Children have been born weighing 13 or 14 lbs., but this is quite exceptional.

How much will a child increase in weight in a given time? The answer to this question will depend to a great extent upon: (1) Whether the child is healthy; (2) Whether it is able to digest its food; and (3) Whether it gets the proper kind of food. Roughly speaking, a baby doubles its weight by the fifth month, and trebles it at the twelfth. It may gain at the rate of 1½ ounces a day for some months together, but this is certainly above the average.

Table I. may be taken as an average increase in weight in the case of a baby weighing 7½ lbs. at birth, and brought up on good breast milk. Table II. shows the average increase in one brought up improperly on cow's milk, starch food, pap, etc.

	Table I.		Table II.	
	lbs.	oz.	lbs.	oz.
At birth	7	8	7	8
,, 14 days	7	14	7	10
,, 3 months	12	8	11	10
,, 6 ,,	15	8	13	10
,, 9 ,,	18	7	17	7
,, 1 year	21	10	18	7

Or again, suppose the baby weighs 6½ lbs. at birth,
the increase should be somewhat as follows :—

				TABLE I.		TABLE II.	
				lbs.	oz.	lbs.	oz.
At birth	-	-	-	6	8	6	8
,, 14 days	-	-	-	6	13	6	10
,, 3 months	-	-	-	9	5	9	0
,, 6 ,,	-	-	-	12	11	10	7
,, 9 ,,	-	-	-	14	4	11	9
,, 1 year	-	-	-	16	7	13	2

The above tables are partly taken from Gerhardt, but
have been modified from later cases. A child reared by
hand and fed with suitable food, will thrive better and
far outstrip one fed exclusively on poor breast milk.
On the other hand, it must be constantly borne in mind,
that for " getting on," nothing can by any possibility
equal good breast milk.

WEIGHING BABY.

Every mother should possess a pair of scales sufficiently large to weigh baby. An infant's weighing
machine is now made with a basket to hold the child,*
which is very convenient. Many monthly nurses, and
mothers too, have a strong dislike to this proceeding,
considering it unlucky and hurtful. Such prejudices
are now, however, becoming things of the past.

The best way to perform the operation is to place the
scales in front of the fire at bath time. A small cushion,
or pillow, should then be placed in the scale pan to
support baby's head, and a warmed flannel pinned
round the naked child, who is then gently placed in the
scales. It is well to put on sufficient weights beforehand
to approximately reach the sum expected, thus saving
time and shortening a proceeding that baby is at all
times apt to resent. Properly managed, the whole
thing can be done under a minute. Of course, the
pillow and flannel must be weighed afterwards, and
their sum deducted from the gross weight.

---

* T. Hawksley, 357, Oxford Street, London, is the maker of these machines, and
he also has weight charts.

The most satisfactory plan is to weigh baby regularly once a week or fortnight, and to keep a chart for reference.

It is astonishing how a few days' diarrhœa or sickness will affect the weight.

If, for several weeks together, baby's weight does not progress satisfactorily, some change in diet is almost certainly necessary. Weight, however, is not everything, for a child may be getting very fat and putting on weight most satisfactorily, and yet be in a very unhealthy condition.

During the first week of its existence a baby rarely increases in weight, but often actually diminishes. This is most marked the first two or three days, after which it may gain a little, so that, at the end of the week, it may weigh the same as at birth. A fair weekly increase may be taken as 6 to 7 ounces. In the case of twins, both are usually rather under size and weight, and often one is much smaller than the other.

PREMATURE BABIES.

Of course, if baby be born prematurely, *i.e.*, before the ninth month, it will almost certainly be under weight, and, if much before its time, will be very small and difficult to rear. It speaks volumes for the care and watchfulness of a mother or nurse who has successfully reared a baby born at seven months. Such a child will probably weigh about 3½ or 4 lbs., and an eighth month baby about 4 or 5 lbs. An infant weighing under 3 lbs. will not probably be long for this world.

Incubators or mechanical nurses are always employed in hospitals, consisting of a sort of glass box, in which the child lives, the temperature being kept up by hot-water pipes or bottles. The results with incubators are very good—the Maternité in Paris giving the following :

Baby's Weight.	Died.	Lived.	Total.
2 lbs. 3 oz. to 3 lbs. 5 oz.	28	12	40
3 ,, 5 ,, ,, 4 ,, 6 ,,	35	96	131
4 ,, 6 ,, ,, 5 ,, 7 ,,	11	101	112

A very tiny baby requires special attention from the moment of its birth. It should be placed in a bath of hot water (temperature 104°) before the fire and washed whilst in the water, and be then wrapped up in a warmed flannel, gentle drying being done without uncovering the child.

A previously prepared coat of cotton wadding with holes for the arms should next be applied, and strips of wadding be wound gently round the arms and legs. The diaper must be placed inside the layer of wool. Over this coat should be placed more wool, and finally a soft woollen shawl (Shetland if possible). The child should be placed in its cradle between warmed blankets, which, with the exception of a small opening for breathing, must entirely envelop it. Hot bottles should be placed on each side and at the feet of the infant, taking care that two or three folds of blanket protect it from being burnt. The air of the room must be kept warm and pure.

The heat of the child must be maintained night and day by filling the bottles with hot water as soon as they become chilled. No nursing should be allowed, except for the necessary changing, which should be done as seldom as possible. In about a week the wadding must be changed, and, if strong enough, another hot bath may be given. If too weak to suck, the milk must be drawn off by a breast-pump into a warmed glass, and feeding managed by a spoon or pipette every hour or two. If no breast milk is available, half this mixture should be given every hour or hour and a half by means of a pipette.

Fully peptonized Milk	2 drachms	
Barley water	5½ ,,	
Milk sugar	¼ ,,	or 15 grains
Cream	½ ,,	

Quality and quantity can be cautiously increased after a week or so, and raw meat juice may with advantage replace the peptonized milk in two or more meals each day.

In France, and now more frequently in England, such infants are often fed by " gavage," *i.e.*, by passing a soft rubber tube down the throat connected with a funnel, into which the food is gently poured. Oftentimes brandy is necessary. At the end of about six weeks, if the child has got on well, it may be treated as an ordinary baby, but will require special care for months, or even years.

Premature children will, of course, be backward in teething, walking, etc.

HEIGHT.

What height ought baby to be? Here again babies vary very much. The average height at birth is 19 or 20 inches.

Just as proper food has its effect on the weight, so has it also on the height. Table I. shows the average increase in height of a baby brought up on good breast milk, and, when weaned, brought up on proper food; by its side is shown the height of one brought up on improper food.

	TABLE I.	TABLE II.
Birth - - - -	20 inches.	20 inches.
6 months - - -	27 ,,	25 ,,
1 year - - - -	31 ,,	27 ,,
4 years - - - -	37 ,,	35 ,,
6 ,, - - - -	43 ,,	41 ,,

The above is only an average; a child of tall parents will, in all probability, be taller than one of short parents, and *vice versa*. A good instance of the influence of the size of parents upon their offspring is seen in the case of the Nova Scotia giantess, whose baby weighed 23¾ lbs. and was 30 inches long.

HEAD AND CHEST.

In new-born infants, the greatest circumference of the head is more than that of the chest taken just below the nipples. At a year and a half or two years the two measurements should be about equal, after which time the chest increases in size much more rapidly than the head.

5

	Head.	Chest.
3 days old - - - - -	$14\frac{1}{4}$	$13\frac{1}{2}$
6 months - - - - -	17	16
1 year - - - - -	18	$17\frac{3}{4}$
2 years - - - - -	$18\frac{3}{4}$	$18\frac{3}{4}$
4 ,, - - - - -	$19\frac{3}{4}$	$20\frac{1}{3}$
12 ,, - - - - -	$20\frac{1}{2}$	24

The above are only approximate, but it should be noted that in ill-developed children the chest measurement may not exceed that of the head at six or seven years old.

Undue enlargement of the head occurs in rickets and in water on the brain.

CHAPTER VIII.

WHERE SHALL I PUT BABY?

Suffocation—The Cradle and Bassinette—Bed Clothes—Nursery
—Night Nursery—Ventilation—Pure Air—Cubic Space—
Temperature—Cleanliness—Drainage—Quarantine—Infection
—Disinfection.

SOME years ago it was always thought that, for at
least the first month of its life, a baby should sleep
in its mother's bed. This was a very bad habit, for the
child breathed hot, impure air, and it very often led to
too frequent feeding. Sometimes, too, the terrible
accident of suffocation happens from the mother during
sleep pressing the infant too closely to her, or partially
turning over upon it. Sixteen hundred deaths from
this cause alone occurred in England and Wales in 1902.
This danger has been properly recognized in Germany,
and there it is illegal for a young infant to sleep with an
adult.

THE CRADLE OR COT.

From the very first day of its life a baby should have
its own little bed, bassinette, or cradle. Unless standing
high of itself, it should be placed on two chairs to keep it
from draughts.

It should be lined, and have curtains at the head, and
should contain a mattress, a soft pillow with a fine calico
or linen pillow-slip, an under blanket, a pair of soft top
blankets, and a knitted or eiderdown quilt. No sheets
are needed.

As shown elsewhere, *wool* is the best warmth-retaining
material that there is, and babies need this in a very
great degree. If the weather be very cold, an india-
rubber or stone hot-water bottle should be placed in the
cot, but with two thicknesses of blanket between the
child and the bottle. A baby can generally sleep in its

cradle till nine or ten months old, and then a crib should be obtained, made with high sides, which are the same height all the way round, and which, if possible, let down. It should have a woven wire mattress, with a thin hair mattress above it, and be made up in the same way as the cradle. A piece of indiarubber sheeting put beneath the under blanket will protect the mattress. For the sake of appearance a sheet may be put over a blanket, and be turned back over the quilt, which should still be very light. No heavy clothing should ever be found on a child's bed. If expense be a consideration the cradle can be dispensed with, and a small sized iron or brass cot used from the first. The side near the mother's bed can be left down altogether until the child is old enough to turn about.

It is a good plan to stretch netting over the top of the cot to prevent a child standing up and overbalancing. Many broken limbs have been the result of neglecting this important precaution. Nets are sold for the purpose, or can be quickly made by a netter at home with bright colour macramé thread. The bedding and bed clothes should be placed before an open window every day for an hour to thoroughly purify them. On wet days this should be done before a brisk fire.

THE NURSERY.

The Room that a child is to occupy, both in the night and day, must be carefully considered. For the first fortnight of its life baby will probably stay in its mother's room, but afterwards, if it can be managed, it is best to set apart a room for it—the Nursery.

This is the most important room in the house, and should be chosen with care. It should be high up, though not exactly under the roof, face the south or west, and be lofty, for it should abound in air and sunlight, without which it is impossible to rear healthy children.

Wherever possible there should be a night as well as a day nursery, which much simplifies matters of ventilation; but where there is only one child, one room is frequently all that can be given up to it. In the latter case, twice every day the child must be taken into another room, and the doors and windows of the nursery thrown wide open for an hour to change the air in every corner.

Pure Air contains a large amount of oxygen, which we inhale every time we breathe, exhaling at the same time carbonic acid gas. Oxygen is essential to life, whilst carbonic acid gas is poisonous. It will thus readily be seen that in a room filled in the morning with pure air, and inhabited all day by persons taking in the oxygen, and replacing it by carbonic acid gas, unless the room be well ventilated the air will become more and more impure, until at last it is positively dangerous to life. Many babies have lost their frail little lives from lack of this knowledge on the part of their parents. Therefore, if a child is to inhabit the same room as its parents by day and night, it follows that very great care will have to be taken to keep the air in that room fit for the little one to breathe.

Ventilation.—In order to secure proper ventilation without draught, it is necessary to allow a space of about a thousand cubic feet for each grown-up person. The cubic space of a nursery can easily be found by multiplying its height, length, and breadth together, though, of course, any furniture, especially if bulky, will take up room and make the available space less. Supposing the height of the nursery be 10 feet, its breadth 14 feet, and its length 20 feet, that would give $10 \times 14 \times 20 = 2,800$ cubic feet, which would be ample for a nurse and two children.

Although a nursery be quite large enough, there must, at the same time, be proper ventilation. What is proper ventilation? It is an adequate change of air without draughts, and for this it is necessary to have a way for the impure air to go out, and a way for the fresh air to come in. The open chimney, especially when there is a fire, answers for the first, and the opened window for the second.

The window may be kept constantly open without causing a draught, by having a piece of wood, six inches high, nailed to the lower sill in front of the sash. The lower sash is then opened three inches or so. Provided there is no direct draught, the windows should also be drawn down about three inches from the top. Tobin's system of allowing air to enter by shafts, six or seven feet high, placed round the room, is very good. The atmosphere of the nursery can thus be kept fairly pure, but the systematic airing twice a day must still be attended to. In very cold weather, after the airing, the room must be thoroughly warmed before a young baby is re-admitted.

The windows, which should be low so that the children can see out, must be protected inside by railings to prevent accidents ; and a fire, well protected by a guard, is far better than a stove.

A thermometer should be kept in the nursery, and the temperature maintained at about 60° F.

The nursery floor should, if possible, be covered with cork carpet or linoleum, and a large square of carpet be placed in front of the fire-place. There should be very little furniture, and, if it can be managed, another room should be used for the nurse's dressing room, where she can keep her own clothes, baby's washing apparatus, all soiled linen, etc.

The floor should be washed over every week, and dusted every morning.

If the walls can be painted it is the best thing to do, but if not, sanitary wall paper, which can be washed, should be used. Bright coloured pictures should be on the walls, and a swing fastened to a cross-beam is a great amusement.

No Food should be kept in the nursery, especially milk. Slops of all kinds must be removed immediately, as they contaminate the air, which, it cannot be insisted upon too often, must be kept as pure as possible, especially in stormy weather when the children are obliged to remain indoors.

Every intelligent mother will now be able to frame rules for the proper ventilation of the children's living and sleeping rooms, and will, of course, see that the more people there are in a given space, the oftener will the air require to be changed, because the quicker will it get polluted.

Gas burners use up a great deal of oxygen, and should never be kept lighted when the children are asleep. A night light is quite sufficient. Small safety reflector lamps, which leave the room dark except where the light is needed, are very useful.

The Drainage of the house is of great importance, and no pipes should be allowed to enter direct into the main sewer. Untrapped or improperly trapped pipes are a very fertile source of illness, often causing diarrhœa, sore throat, diphtheria, low fever, etc.

ISOLATION AND DISINFECTION.

When a child is suspected of having any infectious disease it should be at once isolated, even before the doctor arrives, for some fevers, *e.g.*, measles, are very contagious at quite an early stage. Quite true, in some cases the child may only be suffering from a bad cold or simple feverish attack ; but no harm has been done, and it is always best to err on the safe side.

If whooping cough or measles break out in a house where there is a weakly baby, it is by far the best plan to send the infant away altogether. Children attacked with scarlet fever had best be sent to hospital, especially if there be other children in the house.

Isolation is always very difficult to carry out thoroughly, but it is of no use to set about it in a half-and-half style.

The best room to choose is one at the top of the house, and, if possible, the whole of the top floor should be given up to the patient and nurse. All superfluous furniture should be removed, including the carpet, window curtains, bed hangings, etc., and a sheet kept continually wet with carbolic acid one in forty, or Jeyes' disinfectant one in twenty, hung up over the doorway.

Of course, the nurse is just as liable to carry contagion as the patient, and should not mix with the family at all.

Minor cooking, *e.g.*, warming up beef tea, milk, etc., should be done upstairs by the nurse, as also the washing up of cups, plates, etc.

All soiled linen should at once be placed in a disinfectant before going to the wash.

The doctor will say when the period of infection is over, and will probably order disinfecting baths. The child and nurse should then have fresh clothes, and the rooms be disinfected. This disinfection is best carried out by the District Sanitary Inspector, to whom application may be made. The usual plan is to shut up the room and burn sulphur or use formalin. After twenty-four hours the door and windows are opened, and the floor scrubbed with carbolic soap.

In cases of scarlet fever the ceiling will require to be white-washed, and the walls stripped and papered.

Chapter IX.

BABY'S NURSE.

BABY must have a nurse—that is certain, and a nurse, too, for a good long time. Baby is not like a puppy, which, in a few days, will begin to act independently, and in a few weeks can dispense with any special looking after. A baby-man or woman develops very slowly, and needs constant supervision, even in the most elementary matters, for the first three or four years of its life.

It has often been said that the best nurse a child can have is its mother, but this is by no means always true.

A good nurse must possess certain qualities, be she the mother of the child or not.

THE NURSE.

If a mother can afford it, and especially if she be young and inexperienced herself, it is better not to choose too young a nurse for her first child ; and she should give the preference to one who has had the care of quite young infants · previously. A good nurse will always gladly learn the best methods of managing and bringing up a child, and should never be above learning from her mistress ; neither should any mother be above learning from her nurse.

A really competent nurse is an unspeakable treasure to a young mother ; but if her views on ventilation, artificial feeding, etc., be erroneous, her ideas must not be blindly followed. A nurse should never be ashamed to confess ignorance, which is far better than to hazard a confident opinion upon a subject of which perhaps she knows nothing.

A good nurse should possess a strong love for children, simply because they are children, and should prefer being a nurse to anything else. A person who has this characteristic, is rarely lacking in the second all-essential quality—that of patience. To lose one's temper with a naughty child is a fatal mistake.

The nurse must also be perfectly trustworthy, obedient, and truthful, or how can she teach these qualities to her charges ? Many a child has had his first lesson in deceit from his nurse saying : " I will give you so and so, if you won't tell,"—or from seeing things done, when the mother is absent, which would not be thought of were she at home. She should be perfectly healthy ; one who is markedly scrofulous or consumptive may act as the innocent cause of a child's ill health or perhaps death.

It may be useful here to mention that nurses are often seen in the streets, parks, and public promenades, ostensibly in charge of children, but who are reading, chatting to other nurses or acquaintances, looking into shop windows, or even doing a little shopping on their own account. Some even go so far as to take their little charges on visits to their friends or relations. Now a person who will do any of these things, except by special permission, is quite unfit to be entrusted with children ; she cares more for herself and her own pleasure than for the little ones under her care. Many a case of bronchitis or fever has arisen through carelessness in one of these respects, and it is wise for every mother to make strict rules on this subject which, if wilfully broken, should lead to dismissal.

Young children should never be taken shopping, if it can possibly be avoided ; but a nurse should always feel that, when necessary for herself, she has only to ask permission, and it will be arranged that she shall go out quite free from responsibility of the children.

A good nurse is, or ought to be, a second mother to

the children, so that, when away, their real mother may leave them in her care with perfect confidence that the welfare of the little ones is in safe keeping. Such a nurse should have her authority always upheld, and if she be perhaps wrong in some little question of nursery discipline, this should be pointed out to her afterwards, and not before the children. Mother and nurse should always act as one, and a nurse should always inform the mother at once should she notice the slightest thing unusual in the children under her care.

Cleanliness, tidiness, and method, are also very important qualities in a nurse.

Cleanliness—in her person, and in every corner for which she is responsible, be it a child's ear or a nursery cupboard.

Tidiness—or otherwise the nursery will soon degenerate into a scene of indescribable confusion. Drawers and shelves should each be in perfect order—a place for everything, and everything in its place.

Method—because, though a muddler may get on fairly well with one baby, when there are several she has "never done," and is always trying to make up time, though, of course, never succeeding in doing so. There is often more comfort in a nursery with four children and one methodical nurse, than with one child and no method.

TRAINING BABY.

The training of a child, whether it be by mother or nurse, cannot begin too early. The popular idea of reserving the training of a child until it can talk, is utterly erroneous.

Infants are creatures of habit, good or bad habits being easily formed, but not at all easily broken. Baby, when only a few days old, may have formed the habit of sleeping beside its mother, and obstinately refuse to go off in its cradle. It may have formed a habit of waking and crying to be fed every hour or two during the night, and yet sleeping three or four hours together during the day. A little later on it may have formed the habit of never going to sleep without being rocked in the arms—a very troublesome habit indeed, when the household has resumed its busy round, and baby is no longer everybody's first thought.

To form good habits in baby is, then, the first step in its moral training, and, as before said, cannot be begun too soon. Good habits are as difficult to break as bad ones.

Sleeping.—Regular feeding has been already mentioned, and is most important, but a few words must be said on " getting a child to sleep." A healthy infant will at first sleep nearly all the twenty-four hours ; it requires very little exercise, *i.e.*, nursing and dancing about, and the quieter it is kept the better. After each meal it ought to be laid in its cradle, whether asleep or awake. It should be a rule that, after each meal baby should lie down for at least half-an-hour, and be left quiet.

For the first seven or eight months the child, if treated in this way, will generally take a long or short sleep, just as it feels inclined, after each meal. A child made to lie in its cradle except when being fed, taken out of doors, or occasionally nursed, will very rarely give any trouble when bed-time comes. When sleepy, it will go to sleep, and when wakeful, it will lie and kick about and coo to its heart's content, taking far more exercise, and being just as happy, as though always being nursed. The child will thus form a habit of loving its cradle, instead of hating it as so many do. Never accustom a child to being rocked to sleep, and never wait by its bedside while it is settling off.

Sometimes of course a baby is chilly, either from careless bathing, or exposure, and then it would be cruel to put it down in a cold cradle,—wrap it up in a blanket, and thoroughly warm it by the fire, and then it will go off happily enough. Never forget the grand rule of putting a child into its cradle directly after each meal.

Cleanliness.—Next to good habits in feeding and sleeping, comes the good habit of cleanliness. Here, again, everything depends upon regular perseverance. The child should be systematically held over a utensil before a fire when being changed, and at two or three months old, immediately after each meal. At this age, the habit of going awake into its cradle will be firmly established, and the little intervening incident will make no difference, so long as it is quickly performed, and the child laid down directly afterwards.

A baby, if healthy and brought up to good habits, is a very contented little creature. Until five or six months old, the pleasure of kicking and playing with its hands and feet is all-sufficient, though it may be increased by a rattle or bright-coloured object being suspended over its cot. After this age, an india-rubber or rag doll will amuse for hours, but the child should not be allowed to sit up to play until nine months old, and then only very occasionally. If tired of lying flat, the child must be well bolstered up with pillows.

Baby Comforters should never be tolerated, and it shows a defect in nursery training when a child in a perambulator is obliged to be pacified with such a device. They are stated on good authority to be one of the chief causes of adenoids. The continual sucking also causes an increased flow of saliva, which is too useful a fluid to be wasted in this fashion. On the other hand, Baby's natural comforter—his thumb—may be permitted in reason, as it will often be only sucked when going to sleep. At about ten or eleven months old, baby will probably learn to crawl, and with a few toys will be good for a long time, especially if it can watch older children at play. Soon after a year old, baby will learn to walk a little, but the exact date for this accomplishment is very uncertain.

TOYS.

Contentment is a great virtue to be cultivated in the nursery, and no good nurse will tolerate continual crying and whining ; indeed, as a rule, they are the result of having nothing better to do. A child will often amuse itself for a long time by running round the table, singing as it goes, and when tired of that will be ready for some toys. A nurse should husband her resources, and should never allow all the toys to be had out at once. It is a good plan to keep certain toys in reserve for wet days, *e.g.*, a doll's cradle with its bed-clothes and doll inside, or a set of tea things, with scraps of chocolate and sugar.

Most children, as soon as they can run, enjoy toys which they can push or pull about after them ; strong unpainted playthings which will bear rough treatment are the best. Children like to imitate their elders, and a needle and cotton with a small piece of flannel will amuse for a long time, if only allowed occasionally. A pencil and paper, or large glass beads to thread, are always a source of delight, and, a little later, some Kindergarten toys should be provided. From a farm-yard or Noah's ark, a child will soon be able to pick out the animals correctly. Celluloid toys should be avoided, as they are highly inflammable. Picture books are a great delight ; but until he can be taught to turn over the leaves carefully, they should always be shown by some one, or the child will become destructive. Pictures should always be of a pleasing character, and true to nature, for a child should never have to unlearn what it has once learnt. In teaching the name of objects, it is far better to give the true name at once, *e.g., horse*, not *gee-gee : dog*, not *bow-wow*. As the child gets a little older, it is confusing to know the same object by two different names.

A child should always be taught to put away one set of toys before bringing out another, and little dots of eighteen months will soon learn what tidiness means. The nursery should be a happy place ; of course, every child likes to come downstairs to its parents, but, if the nurse be a true mother, it will be just as ready to go back again.

LESSONS.

A child for the first four or five years should learn simply by object lessons, and will thus lay the foundation for after-study. Simple tales of natural history are always eagerly picked up, but to seriously begin lessons at too early an age is a mistake. All the Wesley family are stated to have been taught their alphabet on the day that they were five years old, but except as a change of amusement, nothing of this kind should ever be insisted on,

Infant schools are a great boon to mothers who are obliged to earn their living, but a good Crèche or Day Nursery is far preferable, and no more expensive. At five or six, a Kindergarten school may be thought of.

If a child be sent to school, it is useless to be always coddling it up and keeping it away for the slightest thing, but the constitutions of children vary, and a delicate one must be specially provided for. Dr. C. Dukes points out that the following three classes of children require to be surrounded by specially favourable conditions during their school life :—

(1). Children who are sickly and delicate.
(2). Children who have had a disease which, under unfavour-able circumstances, will almost certainly recur, *e.g.*, scrofula.
(3). Children who, though healthy, are begotten of parents who have had diseases which are very apt to be trans-mitted to their offspring, *e.g.*, consumption.

MORAL TRAINING.

Children's rules must be few in number, but what there are must always be enforced.

Obedience.—This will entail some struggles, but the child must be brought to see that the mother's or nurse's will is stronger than its own—then, and not before, will it give in. On this point, as indeed on every point, the mother and nurse must act as one ; a child must not be allowed to do a certain thing downstairs which it is forbidden to do upstairs, or *vice versa.*

The obedience must be that of love, not terror, and a little tact is here of great use. To tell a child not to do a thing is but to create the wish to do it, and is just human nature the wide world over. Do not be content with the negative, always suggest something positive ; forbid a child to open a drawer and, at once, it will begin to be restless and fidget about, and at length will proba-bly go up and open it. But if the prohibition be accompanied by a positive request, *e.g.*, to fetch mother's thimble, the difficulty will be over ; the desire to open the drawer will be forgotten, and will consequently vanish.

Direct disobedience should never be overlooked ; but

never as punishment deprive a child of its food, or shut
it up in the dark.   Taking away anything it is very fond
of, *e.g.*, a favourite doll or toy, will be acutely felt.   Being
made to sit quietly on a stool for ten minutes is another
good method.

In very extreme cases, *e.g.*, an act of direct spite or
cruelty, a sound slap may be required, but should only
be administered by the parent.   Never box a child's
ears.   Parents when obliged to punish, should always
make the child feel how grieved they are to be forced
to do so, and that it is not inflicted in the spirit of
revenge.   Favouritism should be carefully guarded
against, always remembering that children have a very
keen sense of justice.

A child often passes through a phase in which there is
an extreme dislike to obeying the slightest command,
even in the ordinary events of life, but it is as a rule only
temporary.

Should he, for example, absolutely refuse to be dressed
to go out, take no notice of the refusal, but while beginning to button his shoes talk away of the little ducks he
is going to feed in the park, or remind him of the game
of hide and seek he loves, so that by a lively recollection
of the past, or anticipation of the future, he will quite
forget the objectionable present.   Should these tactics,
however, fail, it is of no use to lose one's temper.   Give
way pleasantly, saying, " Very well, if Baby will not be
dressed of course he cannot go out, but he will have to
stay all alone in the nursery," and there he must be
resolutely left to realise the necessary consequence of
his wilfulness.   A good fit of crying will probably result,
but the lesson will be thoroughly learnt.

A mother should remember that when a child has
lost his self-control it is useless to reason with him.   He
should be left absolutely alone till he is good, wholesome
neglect being too little understood and practised in
many nurseries.

Truthfulness.—A child must at all times be encouraged
to tell the truth.   Never mind what he has done wrong,
let the little one always find in his parent or nurse a
friend to whom he can confess and tell everything.   To

punish a child when he comes to confess a fault, is but to set a premium on telling a lie. Let him clearly see your sorrow for the wrong deed, but do not punish. Many a child has been driven to tell a lie from fear of the consequences of telling the truth. A tiny child will say " yes " or " no " just as it feels inclined, not really knowing the difference, but of course this is an entirely different thing to telling a lie.

Loving-kindness.—This includes a great deal. It is necessary primarily in the parents and the nurse, and the example shown by them of uniform loving-kindness, under the most trying circumstances, goes a long way in teaching it to the little ones. The elder should always share with the younger, but the younger ones must not have the best of everything.

Never allow a child to snatch from anyone ; teach it to ask nicely for a thing, and if baby takes away an elder child's toy, the latter should be taught to give baby something in exchange for its own property.

Never allow a child to cherish a spirit of revenge. How often, if he falls down, is he told to " Whip the naughty floor or chair," as the case may be, or even allowed to vent his wrath upon some naughty person who displeases him. No ; tell the child to " Kiss the place and make it well," or rub in a little Eau de Cologne, and he will be pleased and quite forget to be angry.

Of slight falls and knocks it is best to take no notice ; too much sympathy engenders a fretful disposition, easily upset by trifles. Gentleness and loving-kindness to all living creatures should be insisted upon.

There is a great difference between animal spirits and rowdiness. It shows a painful want of training, for children always to rush into the sitting-room, slam the door, and stamp on one's toes in their wild spirits. A lack of reverence is very noticeable in the youth of the present day, and respect for elders should be early enforced.

The nervous system of a child should receive a great deal of attention from quite early days. It is exceedingly sensitive, *i.e.*, it responds instantly and intensely to any outside influence, and if stimulated unduly, many serious troubles may arise. For this reason a young child should not be constantly played with or talked to. When awake it should lie quietly in its cot or on a sofa, where it can watch people moving about, and outside impressions can be received slowly, as the nervous system can bear it. A precocious child is one to be dreaded, and to be kept especially quiet, and *never* have its sayings or doings repeated in its presence, much less be encouraged to perform before admiring visitors.

A child should never be frightened, and stories of ghosts, bogies, fire, and robbers should be left untold. Ugly sights and discordant noises, *e.g.*, Guy Fawkes and Punch and Judy shows, strongly affect some children, and should then be avoided for a time, gradually training the child to calmness and self control in the presence of strange sounds. In these children a sudden terror has produced fits, or St. Vitus' dance, or has caused a shock from which the child has never really recovered.

Night Terrors, where a child awakes crying with fright, have often their origin in *days* of excitement. Never hold up the doctor as an object of fear, it will create in the child's mind a spirit of distrust and a horror of all medicines.

Usefulness and Tidiness.—These are important items in a nursery education. All toys should be put away by the children themselves, and it is astonishing how tidy a child of two years old may become, even putting away things that its mother may have left about. A child delights to be made useful ; to fetch and carry little things from one room to another, to fetch its father's slippers, or mother's gloves ; to pretend to dust the furniture,—all these things and many more go to make up a great deal of happiness for a child, and, at the same time, teach it many useful lessons.

It will thus be seen that moral training requires much wisdom. A spoilt child is a nuisance to itself and everyone else, and a lasting monument of disgrace to its guardians.

SICK CHILDREN.

A few words must be added on the subject of nursing sick children.

Children's hospitals are the places where the art of nursing the little ones is to be seen almost in perfection, and, in any very serious illness, if the parents be poor, the kindest thing is to take their children there. In many cases, if it can be afforded, a trained sick-children's nurse will prove a great help, and, in some special cases, is almost indispensable.

It is in illness that a wise mother will reap the benefit of her careful training in good habits.—sleeping, feeding, obedience, etc. A sick child requires a great deal of "letting alone." The quieter it is kept in its cot, not dandled in the arms, the better. The struggles of a spoilt child over taking its medicine or food, have often gone a long way towards causing a fatal termination. In nursing sick children, there must be infinite patience, but invincible firmness; a vast amount of tact, but absolute truthfulness. If something nasty has to be swallowed, there should be no saying: "Now, darling, will you take something nice?" Once deceive a child, and it will never trust you again. Truth is essential; to say—"Now, darling, you must take this, it is not very nice, but will make you better, and you shall have a piece of chocolate after it," is far better policy, and will nearly always succeed with a child who has been brought up to obey.

Should the child refuse, do not worry and irritate it, but lift it gently out of bed, wrap a sheet several times round it, with the hands by the sides, gently hold its nose, and, when the mouth opens, put the spoon containing the medicine as far back as possible, keeping it there until the fluid be swallowed. This may, in some cases, apply to feeding. There must be no sign of anger or impatience on the nurse's part, but the operation should be performed just as a necessary consequence of the refusal on the child's part to take food or medicine. It will not often require repetition.

The strength of a child should be carefully husbanded. If ordered to bed it should be kept lying down, and, if

really ill, other children excluded. Reading or relating
little histories of its every-day life are usually great
charms to a child.

The nurse of a sick child cannot go on continually
without being relieved, as one who is overwrought and
tired out cannot be cheerful and patient. A competent
person must take duty while the nurse has exercise or a
night off duty.

In serious cases of illness it is always well to keep a
chart, and note down every time the patient takes food,
sleeps, has the bowels open, etc., for example :—

6.0 a.m.	- · -	took 4 oz. of milk.
8.0 ,,	- - -	,, 6 oz. ,,
9.0 ,,	- Temperature 103° ;	took medicine.
10.30 ,,	6 oz. of beef tea ;	bowels open.

This acts as a guide to the doctor as well as to the nurse.

A sick child is soon up and down, and, when on the
road to recovery, often traverses it with rapid steps.
Convalescence is often a more trying time to the nurse
than any. A new picture book, or some Kindergarten
work to employ the hands, is now called for ; but, as a
general rule, a child recovering from a severe illness will
sleep a great deal more than when in health. This is
one of nature's methods of renewing the waste to which
the tissues have been subjected, and should be encouraged as much as possible.

The Sick Room, except in some cases of brain and eye
disease, should always have plenty of light and fresh air.
In fever cases, the room requires special treatment.
elsewhere described.

Chapter X.

BABY'S TROUBLES.

IT will now be well to consider some of the minor
troubles which baby may, at one time or another,
be called upon to endure ; for an infant, however healthy,
is subject to little ailments which every mother should
be prepared for and know how to treat.

VACCINATION.

The object of vaccination is to protect the child from
small-pox.   Many mothers have very strong objections
to having their children vaccinated, which they base
on the following grounds :—

(1). It pains the child.

(2). It may introduce diseases, and even cause death.

(3). It is quite unnecessary, and practically of no
value.

Now, the operation itself is hardly painful at all,
especially if care be taken that the arm do not bleed,
and the younger the child the less it is disturbed by the
after effects.   Some children " take " much more than
others, and so suffer more afterwards, but it is rare for a
child to be upset for more than a day or two.   As to the
introduction of disease, this practically never happens,
and could only arise through great want of care.   That
it is valueless can hardly be maintained in the face
of facts.   Indeed, we now hardly know what small-pox

is. The value of vaccination is amply demonstrated by
the fact that no nurse or attendant in the Small-pox
Hospitals ever takes the disease, because efficiently
vaccinated.

The following statistics are taken from the Small-pox
Hospital :—

Of every 100 persons admitted 35 per cent died who
had never been vaccinated, 4 per cent died who had
two vaccine scars, while only 1 per cent died who had
four vaccine scars.

Should vaccination ever be postponed ?—Certainly.

(1). If the child has a skin eruption, *e.g.*, eczema.

(2). If the child be in a state of ill-health.

(3). If the child have recently had an illness.

Vaccination is supposed to have been performed by
three months after birth, and in any case should be
well over before teething begins. It is, however, a
very usual custom now to vaccinate babies at about
a month old or even earlier. In some Maternity Hospitals the babies are vaccinated when a few days old—
and with most happy results—the small patients appearing to take no notice whatever of the proceeding, and
as they move about less at an early age, there is less
irritation.

It is usual to vaccinate in three or four places, high up
on the arm, taking care that the insertions are not too
near together, or they will run into each other and produce a large sore. If the operation be successful, a
small red pimple will be observed on the third day, at
each insertion ; on the fifth day the red pimple turns
into a spot, with a watery head. This spot slowly
enlarges, and the skin around it becomes red, hot, and
tender. About the tenth day the place bursts and
discharges, whilst the centre dries up into a black scab,
which falls off on about the twentieth day, leaving a
depressed scar. An arm that is not practically well
by three weeks should have medical attention.

The child usually suffers most from about the eighth
to the eleventh day, and may be slightly feverish, off
its food, and restless. The amount of pain, however,
varies very much, many children not suffering at all.

It is of importance that the places are not subjected to friction, or violence of any kind, otherwise the spots will get broken, or have their tops knocked off before the proper time. Many mothers use vaccination shields, but they are usually most inefficient, and apt to get out of place, thus creating the very evils they are meant to avert. A pad of antiseptic gauze can be fastened on about the eighth day, and be left undisturbed. Some doctors paint the sites of inoculation as soon as dry with some impervious solution, *e.g.*, zinc gelatine, which forms a protective covering, and enables the child to have its bath as usual.

Erysipelas is a rare complication of vaccination, and is usually due to a want of cleanliness. It is no uncommon thing for a rash to appear within a few days, but it is only of a temporary nature.

Does it matter in how many places a child is vaccinated? Yes. One mark does not protect as well as two, or two as well as three. Three good marks may be considered quite satisfactory.

Will one vaccination protect an individual for a life time? Well, as time goes on, the effect passes off, and it is better to be revaccinated at ten and again at twenty-five. In Germany, where compulsory vaccination and re-vaccination are thoroughly enforced, small-pox is practically unknown.

TEETHING.

The date at which the first tooth appears is very variable. Children have been born with teeth, whilst, on the other hand, the first may not appear until the child is more than a year old.

An acute illness will delay teething, but the chief cause of late dentition is rickets.

The order in which the teeth should be cut is as follows :—

About the seventh month the two middle teeth in the lower jaw. A few weeks later the two middle teeth in the upper jaw ; these four being the central incisors.

At eight months the lateral incisors, top and bottom.

At twelve months the four back teeth or molars.

At sixteen months the four eye teeth.

At twenty-four months the other four molars.

The above constitute the temporary or milk teeth. If not cut in the right order baby is said to cut its teeth " cross."

Most healthy children cut their teeth with very little trouble, indeed the teeth are often through before the mother is aware that anything is going on.

When teething, the gum becomes swollen and hot, and the child will dribble a great deal and put its fingers in its mouth. Here it might be mentioned that without care this constant dribbling may be a source of danger, through the child's clothes becoming saturated, the consequent chilliness producing bronchitis. A jaconet bib should be worn beneath the ordinary one—jaconet being a thin cloth faced on one side with mackintosh. Beneath the gum can often be seen the white line of the coming teeth.

Some children cut their teeth with difficulty, getting an attack of eczema, bronchitis, or diarrhœa with each tooth. The eye teeth are often more trouble than any of the others.

Whilst teething a child should be specially guarded against catching cold.

If the tooth seem nearly through, the gum may be gently rubbed with the end of a thimble or an ivory ring.

Sometimes, when cutting a tooth, the child will get very fractious and restless, waking up many times during the night, starting and screaming. A little bromide is often very useful in these cases. A warm bath, also, given as follows, is often most soothing :—

Put water of temperature 105° into a bath of sufficient depth to reach to the child's waist when sitting down. Place a board or sheet over the bath for the child's toys, and keep it in five minutes, not allowing the hands or any part above the waist to be wetted. A little shawl should be fastened round the upper part to prevent chill. When taken out the lower part of the child will be of a scarlet colour, and it should be well rubbed and put to bed.

Convulsions during Teething are not very common. A hot bath and a dose of castor oil is the best treatment, and the tooth may need lancing. It is a pity to lance a tooth too early, as the point will then have difficulty in piercing through the scar. A slight diarrhœa may act as a safety valve during teething, but it should never be allowed to become at all severe, or it will quickly weaken the child.

How soon should a child's teeth be cleaned ? As soon as it has any. The mouth washing with the finger wrapped in linen having been regularly carried out twice a day from birth, a soft tooth brush can be substituted as soon as the eight incisors are cut. A little good soap may be used occasionally.

It is a great mistake not to carefully look after the milk teeth, as upon their welfare depends, at any rate to some degree, the welfare of the permanent set.

The Permanent Teeth should be cut in the following order :—

Seventh year, four first molars or grinders.
Eighth year, four central incisors.
Ninth year, four lateral incisors.
Tenth year, four first bicuspids.
Eleventh year, four second bicuspids.
Twelfth year, four canine or eye teeth.
Thirteenth year, four second molars.
Seventeenth to twenty-fifth year, four third molars or wisdom teeth.

The temporary set consists of twenty teeth, the permanent set of thirty-two.

If a tooth be at all decayed the child should be taken at once to a dentist, as it should be " stopped " before it begins to ache. It is a very common thing for teeth to be too near together, or too far apart. A dentist should always be consulted in such cases.

FEVERISH ATTACKS.

Nearly all babies at times are subject to these. The nervous system of a baby is delicate to a degree, and that which would not in the least affect an adult may, in an infant, produce a bad feverish attack. In some instances the cause is easy enough to detect; the child is cutting a tooth, has caught a cold, etc.; but very often the cause is so slight as to escape detection; no doubt there is one, but what it is, is unknown.

The signs of a feverish attack are as follows :—The child is off its food, is restless and irritable, the skin is dry and hot, especially the head, which often feels burning, the breath is short and quick, and the pulse beats very fast.

The child should be kept quiet and away from other children, as it is very sensitive to noise, and will probably start at the least sound.

If the bowels be confined, a teaspoonful of castor oil may be given; and if exhausted or restless the child may have, according to age, twenty, thirty, or forty drops of brandy in a tablespoonful of water, which will often have the effect of soothing and getting it off to sleep.

If the child seem ill give it a hot bath, as described under teething, and put it to bed.

It is of no use to press it with food, it will only induce vomiting. For the thirst, milk and water, or barley-water, may be given. It is astonishing how quickly a child will " take a turn " ; one hour it may be lying exhausted, with hot flushed cheeks and a burning skin, panting, and tossing to and fro in its restlessness, whilst the next it may be calmly dozing with a cool moist skin, and sucking its thumb in contentment.

Yet remember that almost all illnesses begin with more or less fever, and what at first may have been taken as " only one of baby's feverish attacks " may afterwards turn out to be the beginning of a long and serious illness.

Temperature.—The amount of fever can easily be ascertained by means of a clinical thermometer. Every mother of a family should possess one, and know how to use it. This instrument is exactly on the same principle as an ordinary nursery or bath thermometer, but on a smaller scale, and contains an index, the top of which marks the highest point to which the mercury has risen. The natural body heat is $98\frac{1}{2}$ degrees (Fahrenheit). This mark on the scale of the thermometer is usually noted by an arrow. The way to take the temperature of a child is as follows :—

Shake down the index of the thermometer until it is below the arrow mark, then draw the arm away from the side and put the bulb of the thermometer well up into the arm-pit, then hold the arm close against the side of the chest for five minutes ; on removal the top of the index will mark the temperature. It is sometimes more convenient to take the temperature in the fold of the groin ; the thigh should in this case be bent up so as to bury the instrument in its crease. Care must be taken that no article of clothing intervene between the skin and the thermometer, and that the instrument do not shift from its proper position. Sometimes the temperature is taken by introducing the bulb of the thermometer into the lower end of the bowel ; the reading will then be about a degree higher than that taken on the surface of the body. The price of a clinical thermometer is about three shillings.

A slight cold will often send the temperature of a child up to 102° or 103°. In bronchitis it often rises to 103° or 104°. But temperature in children has not the same importance that it has in adults ; a child may be 104° and then in a few hours be only 100°, though persistent high temperature indicates disease.

Pulse and Respiration.—Both of these usually have a certain relation to the temperature, *i.e.*, if the temperature goes up, the pulse and respirations will increase in number, and *vice versa*.

Sleep is by far the best, indeed it is the only reliable time to count the pulse and breathing, both of which are at a much higher rate than in an adult. At birth the pulse rate is about 150 to the minute. During the first year it keeps above 100 ; during the second and third years it keeps at 100, or rather under ; during the fourth year 90, and during the fifth 80.

The Pulse of a child can easily be counted, as in the adult, by feeling the number of beats of the artery which is at the front of the wrist, about two inches above the root of the thumb. For a young child another convenient way is to watch or feel the beating of the pulse in the brain at the anterior fontanelle, or hole in the skull. The fontanelle gradually lessens in size, and should be quite filled in by about two years old.

The normal Breathing of an infant a month old is about forty to the minute ; at two years old thirty ; and at eight years old about twenty. The least thing will send up either the rate of breathing or the pulse at once, but no amount of restlessness or excitement will raise the temperature much above the normal. An increase in temperature always means fever.

INFLUENZA COLD.

Infants are very liable to contract heavy colds ; their skins are so sensitive and their whole being so delicately constituted, that they are very susceptible to changes of temperature. The mucous membrane of a child is specially apt to spread a cold, *e.g.*, a cold in the nose or throat is far more likely to spread down the bronchial tubes to the lungs in the case of an infant, than in an adult. Anything that lowers a child's vitality, renders it more liable to catch cold.

A child's vitality may be lowered by insufficient food and warmth, but the most frequent cause is bad air, *i.e.*, air which has been breathed over and over again. On a wet or damp day, perhaps, several children are kept shut up in a nursery all day long with the windows and doors closed. Of course, in a few hours, all the pure air will have been used up, and then they will be breathing over and over again the same air charged with noxious gases. The following day being fine, but damp, the children are sent out of doors, and catch cold. If they had been turned out of the nursery for half-an-hour two or three times the day before, and the room thoroughly aired, they would probably have escaped. Another frequent cause of colds arises from a false idea as to " hardening." Whilst a child has very little hair, the skin of the head is just as delicate as the skin elsewhere, and must therefore be protected from draughts. In a room airy but not draughty, no covering is required, but if taken across a landing, with windows open on all sides, as is quite right, a little woollen shawl should be thrown over the head. When nature has provided a covering of hair, no wrap is required.

A child properly clothed will take no harm in passing through draughts, but to remain stationary in a direct draught will probably bring on a cold. The rule to be observed is plenty of fresh air, but no draughts. Acute nasal catarrh being very infectious, a baby should not be kissed or nursed by anyone suffering from this disorder.

A baby's cold usually begins with a running of the nose by day, whilst at night the upper part of the nose is apt to get stopped up with mucus, which prevents the passage of air through the nostrils and causes it to sleep with its mouth open. A bad cold interferes with sucking, which is very noticeable when the child takes its food, and poor baby cannot suck his thumb when going to sleep. He may at the same time be feverish, restless, and have little appetite.

If the weather be cold he must be kept strictly indoors, and at an even temperature of 62° to 64°. The room should be well ventilated and not allowed to get stuffy. On fine days, in summer, the child may be allowed to go out if the outside temperature be 64°. Diet will require little, if any, alteration ; over-feeding is certainly not to be tried. The bowels should be opened once a day, but no strong purgatives should be used. The stuffiness of the nose may be greatly diminished by gently inserting into the nostrils a new camel's hair brush with a little sweet oil, or, better still, some vaseline with eucalyptus oil, a drachm of the oil to an ounce of the vaseline. Grease may also be well rubbed in over the root of the nose. A bath at 105° in front of a fire, the child being entirely under water with the exception of its head, will often help to get rid of a cold. It should be lifted out of the bath into a warm blanket, rubbed dry without being uncovered, and put quickly into a warmed bed.

CONSTIPATION.

This is a trouble to which hand-fed babies are much more liable than breast-fed ones. Should it occur in the latter, there is generally an insufficiency of fatty matter in the mother's milk, and she should drink more rich milk or cream, and may with advantage take oatmeal, porridge, and stewed fruit. In hand-fed babies a lack of fat in their food is the most usual cause. This may arise from the child's food being too weak, or insufficient in quantity, and should be corrected by the Table on page 37. Should it persist, more cream or some Mellin's food added to each bottle, a little salad oil or cod-liver oil given twice a day, half a teaspoonful of manna, or the juice of stewed prunes, may any one of them prove effectual. Some doctors recommend a little phosphate of soda in each bottle, and if barley-water be used with the milk, oatmeal-water may be substituted.

Constant drugging for simple constipation is bad. Some children habitually go two days without an action of the bowels, and are none the worse for it. First try one of the simple remedies, after which, if useless, it may be well to use an enema of two ounces of soapy water with a dessert-spoonful of olive oil. A small piece of soap passed into the lower bowel will often suffice in infants. Some doctors recommend an injection of a teaspoonful of glycerine, or a glycerine suppository, which often answers very well. Over a year old, a baked apple without the skin, or a little stewed fruit, with coarse moist sugar, will effect what is required. The habit should be early formed of making a child " go " at a certain fixed hour every day. For example, every day directly after breakfast the child should be placed in its chair ; it should not, however, be left there more than five or ten minutes, as long-continued strain-ing is apt to cause prolapse of the bowel.

Cod-liver oil every morning is often very successful ; and friction and kneading over the whole of the bowels not only help to strengthen the muscles, but often greatly assist in regulating them. In some children constipation can easily be corrected by means of a compress. A handkerchief, wrung out of warm water, is folded into an oblong of about twelve by four inches, and placed over the child's belly. A piece of oiled silk or pink jaconet, just big enough to overlap it in all directions, is placed over, and the whole kept in place by a turn or two of bandage. The compress should be put on when the child goes to bed, and kept on all night.

If a child strain much, and pass only a little slime and blood, a doctor should be sent for *at once,* as the case may prove a serious one.

THRUSH.

This is a sign that the child is out of health, and is nearly always due to a want of cleanliness. Hand-fed babies are far more likely to be attacked than those brought up at the breast. Sour milk, dirty bottles, and stuffy nurseries are all likely causes of thrush, which, as is only to be expected, is more prevalent in hot weather.

In order for thrush to thrive, the mucous membrane must be in an unhealthy state. The great preventive is cleanliness, *i.e.,* clean bottles and teats, freshly prepared food, plenty of fresh air, and frequent washing of the mouth.

In a case of thrush, three grain doses of bi-carbonate of soda may be given, twice a day, to counteract the acidity, for a child four months old. A dose of castor oil may be given to start with, and the mouth swabbed out with a piece of soft rag, dipped in a solution of boracic acid, after each meal, a fresh piece of rag being used each time. Lastly, the patches should be painted with glycerine and borax four or five times during the day. If suitable weather the child should go out.

THE NAVEL.

The cord or navel string generally falls off about the fifth day. Usually there is no trouble with it, especially if it have been dressed carefully at the beginning ; but sometimes a sore, with proud flesh, is left, which is difficult to heal.

A distinct weakness is in some cases left at the navel, and whenever the child coughs or cries there is a bulging, and a small swelling appears. The treatment for this

is pressure. This is best applied by carefully making
a pad, and after pushing back the swelling, fixing it
over the place with strapping, and then applying the
ordinary binder. It is well to place something hard
in the centre of the pad, *e.g.*, a slice of cork. The pad
thus applied should not be removed for some days,
and then only for a fresh one to be put on. In cases of
large protrusions a proper surgical appliance will
probably be required.

THE EYES.

The eyes of an infant are very subject to inflammation, and require a good deal of attention. Neglect
at birth, cold, or the access of soap into them may, any
one of them, set up inflammation. Any discharge must
be carefully removed whenever it forms. *Vide*
" Ophthalmia."

SNORING.

This bad habit is usually the result of defective
training in early life. It is of the greatest importance
to educate an infant to habitually breathe through its
nose, and not through its mouth. The air, in passing
through the nasal cavities, is warmed and moistened
before reaching the lungs—a simple preventive of colds.
Whenever a child's mouth is seen to be open, unless
indeed it be crying or feeding, it should be gently closed,
and especially is this necessary when laying an infant
down in its cradle for a sleep. If this be neglected the
throat becomes dry and rough, and the tonsils may event-
ually become enlarged, and snoring will probably result.
In some cases a child is unable to breathe through its
nose, and always has its mouth open : there is then an
obstruction to the free passage of air, due either to
enlarged tonsils, or polypoid growths, known as adenoids,
at the back of the nose. The child should be taken to a
surgeon, who will effect a cure.

INCONTINENCE OF URINE.

Some children suffer from wetting their bed even up
to the age of four or five years. Some are simply cases

of bad habit and neglect, but very often the child is not to blame at all. Many a one has been punished for what was no fault of its own. The first thing to do is to have the child examined by a doctor to see that nothing is wrong, as, in many cases, a slight operation will set all right at once.

If the parent be assured upon this point, patient management, assisted by suitable medicine, will almost certainly succeed. Never allow the child to sleep on its back, and, if necessary, prevent it doing so by tying a reel in position over the middle of the spine. Always lift the child the last thing at night, if possible once during the night, and the first thing in the morning.

RUPTURE.

Hernia is not uncommon even in very young infants. A rupture consists of a portion of the intestine which has been forced through the abdominal wall, and can be felt as a lump under the skin. The groin is the most common place for a rupture, although one may appear near the navel.

When the child cries, the rupture will swell up and get larger, whilst on the other hand, if it keep quiet and stop crying it will become smaller and perhaps quite disappear. If the bowel should come down and get nipped in the opening through which it escapes from the abdomen, the child will be in imminent danger. The bowel has become what is called "strangulated"; nothing can pass through it, and unless relieved it will mortify. When a hernia is strangulated it will not go back into the abdomen, vomiting is quickly set up, there is constipation, and fatal collapse will soon set in if nothing be done to afford relief.

If an infant who is known to have a rupture be suddenly seized with vomiting and constipation, send for a doctor *at once ;* never mind whether the rupture appear down or not, appearances are often deceptive. The doctor will frequently be able to remedy the trouble without an operation. The longer a strangulated rupture is allowed to remain unrelieved, the greater the danger to the child. Never, under any circumstances, should a mother be tempted to try and press back the strangulated rupture herself.

No child is too young to wear a truss; directly a rupture is discovered a truss should be worn. If it be allowed to grow up without one, not only will the rupture continually grow larger, but there will always be the danger of its becoming strangulated.

The truss should be worn day and night, and the parent should always be provided with two in case of an accident. Trusses should never be bought except at proper surgical instrument shops; an unsuitable appliance not only does no good, but a great deal of harm. For young children they are made covered with india-rubber, to prevent soiling, and enabling them to be washed. If the truss be taken off for any purpose the mother should always support the hole through which the rupture comes with the hand, else during a sudden movement or cry of the child it may descend.

The skin in the neighbourhood of the truss must be kept scrupulously clean and dry, and be dusted with starch powder, or chafing will ensue. The truss should be considered as an article of clothing, and will then never be overlooked.

If the wearing of a truss be persevered in from birth, it will probably effect a permanent cure, and at the end of about two years may safely be discarded. The great point with children is *never* to allow the rupture to come down; its descent, even once, will undo all the good the past six months' treatment may have effected. If a rupture persists after this age, take the child to a surgeon, who will probably advise an operation for its radical cure.

PROLAPSE OF THE BOWEL.

This is usually produced by great straining, *e.g.*, in diarrhœa or constipation. In this affection the lower part of the bowel comes down after straining, and protrudes from the orifice as a violet-coloured mass. The great treatment is to regulate the bowels. As a rule the prolapse only occurs when the bowels act, and goes back of itself; if it should not do so, wash carefully, apply some vaseline, and use gentle pressure, the child lying on its stomach. If a child be subject to prolapse, the orifice should be supported by pressing the buttocks together whilst the bowels are acting, and he should never be allowed to sit long upon the vessel for fear of straining. In some cases an operation is necessary.

CONGENITAL DEFECTS.

Harelip is a congenital defect, consisting of a split through one side of the upper lip, usually extending into the nose. The child is generally operated on early in life.

Cleft Palate, which is often associated with harelip, consists of a split or division in the palate, so that the nose and mouth form one cavity.

A child with cleft palate has usually great difficulty in taking its food, because as fast as the milk is taken in through the mouth it returns by the nose. The child cannot create the vacuum in its mouth necessary for sucking, and so is unable to be brought up at the breast. It should be seated bolt upright when being fed, and an old-fashioned boat bottle, with a long teat made for the purpose, employed, so that the flow of milk can be regulated by the inclination of the bottle, and no sucking be required. Of course, the mother's milk can be given after it has been drawn off by the breast pump.

Unless great care and perseverance be used, such a child will not get enough food, and will pine away.

Tongue tie is usually a very minor affair, caused by the tightness of the fold of the mucous membrane which binds down the tongue to the floor of the mouth. The child is unable to protrude its tongue properly, and cannot suck freely. The doctor will very soon rectify it.

Club Foot is a permanent turning of the foot in a wrong direction, so that when older, the child will walk on the inside or outside of the foot, instead of on the sole ; the heel is usually drawn up at the same time. Pliable metal splints, carefully applied, will usually effect a cure. Manipulation, *i.e.*, holding the foot in position, combined with rubbing the muscles of the leg and foot, is very useful, and should be employed whenever the splints are removed. The treatment should never be discontinued until the foot is quite well. It is always a great trial of patience, but the parent will never regret the trouble taken.

No child is too young to undergo treatment, indeed, the younger the better. As soon as he begins to walk he will probably require a light iron in the boot for a short time, to prevent the foot returning to its old distorted position. In a few months, however, the iron may probably be discarded. These "irons" are now usually made of steel, and are far lighter and in every way better than the old-fashioned ones. In some cases the leaders of the foot may be so tight and contracted that it becomes impossible to get the limb into a proper position without dividing them. This is a very trivial operation, and the little puncture made heals up in a day or two.

The great requisite for treating club foot is patience. It is of no use to be in a hurry, and the parent must remember that any bandage, splint, or apparatus, is not to force, but to gradually draw the foot into its right position. A strap or bandage put on too tightly will cause redness of the skin, and, later on, a sore, that may cause treatment to be discontinued some days, and this waste of time has all arisen through being in too great a hurry.

The skin of an infant is exceedingly delicate, and every time the apparatus is changed the limb should be carefully washed, dried, then bathed with a little spirit lotion, and well dusted with starch powder.

Heart disease is usually evidenced by the dark blue colour of the child. A baby may, however, be of a bluish colour for a few days after birth, and then gradually assume a healthy rosy hue, and there may be nothing wrong at all. But if, after a few days, the child still remain blue, a malformation of the heart must be suspected.

Children with congenital heart disease are difficult to rear, any little cold or bronchitis, which in a healthy child would be of no consequence, being of grave import to them, as it gives the heart extra work. In bad cases the skin is of a dark blue colour, and the child pants for breath after the least exertion. Severe cases very rarely live to grow up.

Deaf-mutism.—An infant may be born deaf, and consequently will grow up dumb. When old enough, such a child should be sent to a proper institution, it being almost hopeless to teach it successfully at home. Well carried out lip-reading appears to give the best results.

Idiocy is a form of mental weakness which dates from birth. It varies in degree from a mere feebleness of intellect, to a state in which the mind seems wholly absent. Much can be done by careful training and education, but the child will never be as others.

In the case of poor children it is best to get them admitted into an asylum. For those living in London there is one at Darenth, near Dartford, where they may be admitted between the ages of 5 and 16. The earlier the child is sent the better. In order to gain admission, application should be made to the relieving officer of the parish.

CHAPTER XI.

BABY'S ACCIDENTS.

Accidents — Burns — Scalds — Scorches — Bruises — Concussion — Cuts — Sprains — Dislocations — Fractures — Suffocation — Swallowing Foreign Substances — Choking — Foreign Substances in Ears or Nose — Poisoning — Dog-Bites.

MANY accidents are due to sheer carelessness and neglect ; still, it is a true saying that " Accidents may happen in the best regulated families," and the mother should know what is the right thing to be done in an emergency, and do it at once. It is almost as important to know what should *not* be done, as what to do, for many a trivial accident has been converted into a very serious one by misdirected zeal on the mother's part. The slightest doubt as to what ought to be done, is a clear indication that a doctor should be sent for.

Burns and Scalds are very common among children, especially among the poorer class ; about 3,000 lives are lost every year from these causes. Such accidents often happen through a lighted lamp or a vessel containing hot fluid being upset. Should a child's clothes catch fire, smother the flames with anything handy ; your own dress if nothing better offers. Never wait and call for help, and never carry the child elsewhere, till every particle of flame has been extinguished.

Scalds and burns produce an alarming amount of shock and prostration, especially if the surface involved be large. They are far more dangerous on the trunk than on the limbs. The bigger a burn or scald, even though it be one of slight degree, the more dangerous it is. Whilst waiting for a doctor, cover up the affected parts with soft rags, dipped in sweet oil, and give the child some brandy.

In the case of slight scalds or scorches, a mixture of

equal parts of collodion and castor oil, well mixed together, and applied with a soft paint brush, will allay the pain at once. A solution of carbonate of soda, made as strong as possible, and applied with soft rags, will also quickly give relief.

The course that a bad burn takes may be divided into three stages—(1) *Shock* : this usually lasts one or two days, and is followed by (2) *Inflammation*, which will last about ten days, and be concluded by (3) the stage of *Exhaustion*. During any of these three stages the child may die. Burns and scalds on the chest are peculiarly fatal in young children, as the period of shock is very marked, and inflammation of the lungs is very apt to set in.

If the part be only scorched, fine flour or whitening may be dusted on and covered with cotton wool. If, however, the skin be really burnt, an oily or greasy application will be the best. An ointment of vaseline and eucalyptus oil, or one of boracic acid and lard, spread on strips of lint or linen, should be applied to the affected part, covered by a layer of cotton wool, and kept in position by bandages. Carron oil, which consists of equal parts of olive oil and lime water, is a favourite remedy, but unless it be frequently changed, the odour will not be very agreeable. At first a burn or scald, unless a slight one, will require dressing every day. All should be got ready and the lint spread, before the part be uncovered, so that the wound may be exposed to the air as little as possible. In using lint, the smooth, and not the rough side, should be placed next the skin, or it will stick to the wound and cause needless pain. Blisters require opening about the second or third day. The less often a burn has to be dressed, the quicker it will get well, but then it *must* be kept clean. To know when to dress a burn, and when to let it alone, requires experience.

After the first few days, when changing the dressing, the wound may be cleansed with a little Condy's fluid in warm water. Do not dab the wound, but gently squeeze a sponge full of the lotion, so that a stream trickles over the part.

The pain of a burn is very great, and the dressings will be a great trial to the mother; but the more that antiseptics are employed, the less will be the smell, and the less often will the wound require touching. The antiseptics usually employed are preparations of eucalyptus and sanitas oils, boracic acid, and iodoform.

The general health of the child will require looking after, and convalescence is always very slow.

Burns and scalds always look their best soon after their infliction, and what appears trivial at first is apt about the fourth or fifth day to look more serious. If the skin be burnt through its entire thickness, a scar must ensue; if the whole depth of the skin be not destroyed, there will be no scar. Deep burns, even though small in extent, tend, when healing, to contract and produce deformity, splints being often necessary.

BRUISES, CUTS, AND SPRAINS.

Bruises.—A mother is sometimes unnecessarily alarmed by the sight of a lump on her new-born baby's head. It has formed from pressure during birth, and will probably get all right in a few days. The same cause may in some cases produce paralysis of one side of the face, which will almost certainly pass off after a time.

A child, when beginning to walk, is sure to get a good many tumbles, and probably not a few bruises. A common place for a bruise is the forehead, caused, usually, by the child coming down on something hard, *e.g.*, the corner of a sofa or chair. A tender swelling appears, gradually increasing in size; later on it turns blue, then green and yellow, and finally disappears. If the child seem in pain, put on a little spirit lotion of Eau de Cologne, and a plentiful supply of grease helps to lessen the discoloration. A piece of raw beef applied at once, and changed every hour, is said to cause a bruise to disappear very rapidly.

Concussion.—The skull of a child is very thin, as before stated, and a severe blow on the head should never be lightly regarded. Even though there be no wound or bruise externally, yet the brain may have sustained a shock or concussion. In severe concussion, the child is rendered quite insensible, the breathing is short and quick, and the skin cold. As the effects pass off, the child gets warmer, gradually regains consciousness, and is probably sick. In unfavourable cases, inflammation of the brain may set in, the vomiting may persist, and the case terminate fatally.

In a case of concussion, even if slight, put the child to bed, darken the room, and keep everything quiet. Feed the child very lightly, and, if necessary, give a little castor oil. Quiet and sleep are what the child wants. It is impossible to predict with certainty how such a case may terminate, and a doctor should always be called in.

Cuts.—Children often wound themselves with knives, scissors, etc.; as a rule, a small piece of lint applied to the wound, and kept on until it heals, will set all right. In the case of deeper wounds, where the bleeding will not stop, put on a piece of lint, and bind up very tightly with a long strip of rag, used as a bandage, and the bleeding will probably not recur. But the bandage should be loosened in a few hours, or the part may mortify from the pressure employed.

Sprains usually occur from carelessly lifting a child, or from rough play. The joint may be twisted or strained, becoming swollen and painful. With rest and warm compresses or evaporating lotion it usually soon recovers.

DISLOCATIONS AND FRACTURES.

Dislocations are rare in childhood, and, in such cases, there is always deformity of the joint present. While waiting for the doctor, immerse or bathe the joint in very hot water.

It is not a very uncommon thing for a child to be born with one, or even both hips out of joint. The mother may not detect anything wrong with the child at first, but when walking should begin, something unusual is generally noticed. If the dislocation be single, the one leg will be shorter than the other; if double, the child will waddle like a duck. Some improvement can be effected by operation, and appropriate boots or instruments will help to a great extent.

Fractures.—The commonest fractures which happen to infants are those of the thigh, arm, and collar bones. If the bone be completely broken through, the evidences of the break are generally pretty clear. The child screams with pain on the slightest attempt to move the part, and the broken ends of the bone stick up, forming a lump. Very often, however, the bone is not broken quite through, but is partly bent and partly broken, producing what is called a " green stick " fracture.

" *Green stick* " *fracture* is very common in children, because their bones contain a large amount of fibrous tissue in proportion to the earthy matter, and are thus able to bend without snapping. Fractures in infants generally do very well, if the parts be put up in a suitable apparatus and kept at rest. New bone is thrown out between and round the two ends. This forms a lump, which will gradually disappear as the new bone hardens.

SUFFOCATION.

This accident is not so rare as many think, and usually arises from the mother taking the child to bed with her. It is a common enough thing for a mother to drop off to sleep whilst baby is still at the breast—how probable, then, that she should turn over on the child, and thus suffocate it. There can hardly be anything more heartrending than the feelings of a mother who, on waking, finds her infant dead by her side.

The accident may happen in another way. The infant may be snugly wrapped up in a shawl, and, whilst asleep, partially turn over, burying its face in the wrap ; not having the sense to turn back again, it is suffocated.

In cases of sudden spasm of the air passage, the child may literally die for want of breath, but this is not frequent.

SWALLOWING FOREIGN SUBSTANCES.

At a certain stage, everything that a child can get hold of it puts into its mouth, so that it is a common thing for a child to swallow buttons, coins, small toys,

etc. If the substance swallowed be large, *e.g.,* a crust
of bread, it will stick in the throat, and the child will
get red in the face, put up its hands to its mouth, and
try to cough. The mother should at once put her
finger down the child's throat and try to hook out the
offender. If this do not succeed, and the child
seem on the verge of suffocation, catch hold of it by its
feet and hold it with its head downwards, and give it
a smart smack on the back.

If a foreign body be swallowed, and get safely into
the stomach, the best thing is to do—nothing. Do not
make the child sick ; and, above all, do not give castor
oil or any purgative medicine ; the offending body will
be passed in due time without any further trouble. In
older children porridge and bread and milk form the
best diet, so that a mass may result, in the midst of
which the substance may subsequently be passed without
any injury to the intestine. By giving purgatives the
delicate mucous membrane of the stomach and bowels
will be irritated by the hard offending substance being
rapidly forced along against it.

FOREIGN BODIES IN THE EAR.

Small bodies, *e.g.,* peas, beads, or buttons, easily find
their way into a child's ear or nose. If the substance
be far in, never attempt to extract it ; the child will
almost certainly struggle, and serious results may
ensue. Take the child at once to a doctor, who will,
if necessary, put it under chloroform and extract the
article without any risk or damage. A foreign substance left in the ear will produce permanent deafness.
Ill-advised, bungling attempts to dislodge the offender,
may set up fatal inflammation of the brain.

POISONING.

This is not a common accident in childhood. Many
toys, however, especially those covered with red, green,
or white paint, are poisonous if sucked. Lucifer matches
are poisonous from the phosphorus they contain.
Should a case occur, make the child sick, and send for
a doctor.

A chronic form of arsenic poisoning may occur from the wall paper of the room containing arsenic, and a form of lead poisoning, from water impregnated with that metal.

BITES OR SCRATCHES.

These may occur either by dog or cat, and are apt to cause unnecessary alarm. Should the animal appear to be in its usual health, and have snapped because teased or trodden on, no fear need be felt. The wound should be thoroughly washed with carbolic acid lotion, one part in forty, and dressed with a piece of lint soaked in the same, and covered with a piece of gutta-percha tissue.

On the other hand, should the animal have been morose and off its food for a few days, it should be killed and its body be sent to the authorities, who will examine it, and in a few days inform the sender whether it had rabies, *i.e.*, hydrophobia. Should this be suspected, or the dog be a stray one, the bite should immediately after infliction be strongly sucked, then thoroughly cleaned with a strong solution of carbolic (one part in twenty), and the child be at once taken to a doctor. The immediate sucking to prevent the poison getting into the circulation is most important. If it be proved that the animal had rabies, the doctor will probably recommend treatment by inoculation.

Chapter XII.

BABY'S ILLNESSES.

Illness—Bronchitis—Inflammation of the Lungs—Pleurisy—
Fever—Baths—Wet Pack—Chicken-pox—Measles—German
Measles—Scarlet Fever—Small-pox—Typhoid Fever—Whoop-
ing Cough — Diphtheria — Croup — Laryngismus Stridulus—
Rickets—Skin Affections—Red Gum—Eczema—Nettle Rash
—Ringworm — The Itch — Lice — Worms — Tape Worms—
Round Worms — Thread Worms — Diarrhœa — Dysentery—
Jaundice — Scrofula — Scurvy — Hip Disease— Ophthalmia—
Granular Lids—Ulcer of Cornea—Inflammation of Eyelashes
—Squint—Otitis—Infantile Paralysis—Rheumatism.

I N any case of serious illness the mother should, at the
very beginning, carefully weigh three proposi-
tions :—

(1). Shall I be able to nurse the child myself ?
(2). Will it be best to have a trained nurse ?
(3). Will it be best to send the child to a hospital ?
In order to nurse a child through any serious illness the
mother will have to give up all her time to the patient.
It is useless to think of carrying on the ordinary household duties, while acting the part of nurse. Sometimes,
of course, the question is answered at once in the negative
by the mother being in a state of ill-health, or so delicate
as to be physically unable to withstand the strain; or
she may be suckling an infant. In all cases of serious
illness it is a great comfort to have a thoroughly trained
sick nurse to look after the child. This is more a question
of expense than anything else. A mother, in thus calling
in the services of a trained nurse, must not for a moment
think that she is giving up her privileges, or her duty to
her child. The nurse can do what the mother often
cannot do. It is not only love but knowledge that is
required, and in some cases the mother herself, through
a want of knowledge and training, becomes the chief
obstacle to the child's recovery.

Cases of scarlet fever and diphtheria, unless efficient isolation can be carried out, had better be nursed at a hospital, if there be other children in the same house. With poor people, all serious cases of illness will, with very few exceptions, get well much quicker if sent to a hospital.

It is not a very difficult thing to tell whether a child be ill or not. The loss of appetite, dry skin, and languor, are quickly detected by the watchful mother or nurse, and though, to a casual observer, the child may for a few moments brighten up and appear quite well, the trained eye is not so easily deceived. If a child be very ill, it is always a good sign when it sheds tears; such cases usually recover.

It will be well to consider a little in detail some of the commonest illnesses to which a baby is liable. The following remarks are in no way meant to supersede the doctor, but are given so that the mother or nurse may understand, in some little measure, the nature of the complaint, what course it is likely to take, what are the chief dangers to be feared, and the line of treatment which will probably be adopted.

BRONCHITIS.

By bronchitis is meant an inflammation of the air tubes of the lungs. In certain states of the weather bronchitis may occur in the form of a regular epidemic; cold, wet, and fog are specially conducive to this disease.

Bronchitis is very liable to set in under the following conditions :—

(1). In weak and sickly children.

(2). In rickety children.

(3). As a consequence of an influenza cold.

(4). During attacks of measles and whooping cough.

Inflammation of the smaller air tubes, or, as it is called, capillary bronchitis, is always a dangerous complaint in infants. Bronchitis may begin with an ordinary feverish cold, which gradually spreads downward until it reaches the bronchial mucous membrane. There is always more or less fever, the breathing is quick and short, and at the same time laboured, so that the nostrils dilate with each breath ; the cough is very troublesome, and usually continues during sleep. There is much restlessness and tossing about before the child can find an easy position. The face is often flushed and covered with perspiration. There is a loss of appetite, and often-times sickness. If the child be at the breast, there will be inability to suck properly, on account of the want of breath. Infants rarely bring up the phlegm or mucus which is secreted in bronchitis, in the form of expectora-tion, as grown-up people do, but cough it up into the mouth and then swallow it.

On applying the ear to the back of the chest, wheezing or rattling can generally be heard all over it.

In mild cases of bronchitis, where the larger air tubes are affected, the cough is usually louder, and plenty of air enters the lungs, so that the child, though short of breath, does not pant, turn blue, or dilate its nostrils. The rattling in these cases is louder.

If a child lie quiet, with rapid breathing, blue lips, and a constant little muffled cough, it is very seriously ill indeed.

Good nursing is everything in bad cases of bronchitis. The child should be put into a good-sized room with a fire ; it must be remembered that the little one wants plenty of fresh air, though at the same time it must be warm air. To put the patient into a tiny little bedroom with a roasting fire, is often to take away its only chance. A flannel gown with long sleeves should be worn, as the child is sure to be restless.

The patient may often be quieted by taking him out of bed and nursing him by the fire for a while. A change of position will often afford relief, *e.g.*, turning on to one side, or bolstering up with pillows.

If the child require washing, and is able to bear it, it should be done in front of a fire, with the bath surrounded by a screen. Immerse the child up to the neck in water at 104°, keep it there for three minutes, take it from the bath, envelop it at once in a warm blanket, and dry under it, so that there is no exposure to the air. Next put on the child's garments, wrap it in a warm dry

blanket, and put it to bed with the blanket still around
it.

If the cough be tight and dry, a bronchitis kettle, put
on the fire for a few hours, will often prove of service ; it
will moisten the air and loosen the cough.

If the cough be loose, a kettle is not called for, and
may do harm.   To keep a child in an atmosphere of hot
steam for several days together is certainly a great
mistake. Should the secretion into the bronchial tubes
be abundant, and the child seem almost choked with it,
it is a good plan to induce vomiting, which will clear
off the phlegm and greatly relieve the symptoms.   The
best emetic is a teaspoonful of ipecacuanha wine.

Poultices are much less used than formerly, though
sometimes a jacket poultice made of linseed, with a very
little mustard in it, is ordered at the beginning of the
illness, to be replaced in an hour or so by a hot cotton-
wool jacket.   The great thing to be guarded against is
debility, and the child's strength will require to be kept
up with appropriate nourishments.   Brandy is often
necessary.   Convalescence is often very protracted, and
Kepler's extract of malt, raw meat juice, or cod-liver oil
may be given with advantage.   Even when apparently
quite recovered, the child should not be taken out of
doors until the doctor's sanction is obtained, as a relapse
is very common.

A child that has once had bronchitis, is rather liable to
have it again, and some children cut each tooth with an
attack.   In order to prevent a recurrence of the disorder,
the child must be braced up, and not coddled.   Sun-
shine, pure air by day and night, warm but not heavy
clothing, and an abundance of nourishing food—milk,
cream, eggs, etc.—will render him less susceptible.
Damp cold—not dry cold—is most to be dreaded, and
for town children some weeks in a dry, sunny seaside
place during the foggy season will often prevent an
attack for the whole winter.

INFLAMMATION OF THE LUNGS.

This disease is by itself not a very common one among
young children, being almost always accompanied by

bronchitis, constituting the disorder known as broncho-pneumonia.

In young infants, especially if they be rickety, broncho-pneumonia is very fatal. The treatment is the same as that for bronchitis. Warm, fresh air is required; and to allow several sympathizing friends in to help, and to keep up the warmth of the room by burning gas, is but to deprive the child of the great thing needful, viz., oxygen.

PLEURISY.

This disease consists of an inflammation of the pleura, or covering of the lungs, and, unlike bronchitis, is nearly always confined to one side. After the inflammation has subsided, fluid is very apt to be poured out between the lung and its covering. If this fluid increases to any extent, it will so press on the lung that the child will have great difficulty in breathing, and, unless something be done, will be suffocated. In such cases the doctor will draw off the fluid by sucking it through a hollow needle with a pump.

Sometimes, instead of the fluid being clear, it will be thick, like cream; then an opening will probably have to be made between the ribs, and a drainage tube inserted to allow the fluid to slowly drain away. Usually cases of pleurisy do very well. No doubt it is a terrible thing for the mother to be told that an operation is necessary, and that her little darling's chest must be opened; but consent should never be witheld, it is the best thing to be done, and will in all probability result in a perfect cure.

In all cases of chest disease the child should not be allowed to talk, but be kept as quiet as possible.

FEVER.

Every rise of temperature of the body which reaches a certain height, and lasts a certain time, is a fever. The simple feverish attacks which are so common in young children have been described elsewhere; we now come to the *special* fevers, each of which is caused by its own special poison.

Some fevers are *infectious*, *i.e.*, their poison may be

8

carried from one person to another. Strictly speaking, the word "contagious" means that the disease is spread from one person to another by actual contact, while the word "infectious" means that it is spread without actual contact with the diseased person; but the terms are now often used interchangeably.

Whilst a child is feverish, it is not only useless, but injurious to press it to take solid food. All it wants is to be left quiet, and to be supplied with enough fluid nourishment to allay its thirst.

In cases in which the rash comes out very imperfectly, the child may become very ill. A hot bath is here often very beneficial. The bath should be put in front of the fire, and the child be very slowly let down into it. After being in about five minutes it should be taken out, wrapped in a warm blanket, and put straight to bed without being dried. The temperature of the bath should be 105° F. A bath thermometer should always be used.

When a cold bath is ordered in cases of fever, the child is put into the water at a temperature of about 95° F., and cold water, or even lumps of ice, are added afterwards, till the temperature drops to 60°. Great caution is required whenever baths are used in cases of fever ; the child is sure to be very weak, and dangerous collapse may set in. Brandy should always be at hand in case of necessity. The temperature of a child having a cold bath must be carefully watched, and the doctor or a trained nurse is always present during its administration.

In some cases of restlessness and want of sleep, a wet pack is very useful. The bed is first protected by a mackintosh, with a blanket placed over it. A sheet is then wrung out of hot, warm, or cold water, as the case may be, and the child is enveloped in it, with the exception of its head, and is then placed on the bed, the lower blanket being tucked closely over, and two others laid above. The duration of a wet pack is from half-an-hour to three hours. Besides quieting the child and inducing sleep, the wet pack will bring down the temperature and so reduce fever.

THE INFECTIOUS FEVERS.

Those infectious diseases which are characterized by a rash, are known by the name of " *the exanthemata.*" The word exanthem simply means a skin eruption, but is now exclusively used to denote the rashes or eruptions which accompany the infectious fevers. The most important exanthemata are chicken-pox, measles, German measles, scarlet fever, small-pox, and typhoid fever.

All the exanthemata are more or less contagious ; they all have a period of incubation, *i.e.*, there is a period during which the patient has the poison in his system, although it has not shown itself ; they all possess a rash ; and, lastly, they are all specific, *i.e.*, each is produced by a poison peculiar to itself. It may be useful to give a table of the incubation period of the infectious diseases, as, if after exposure to infection the child does not develop the disease by the time mentioned, it will not do so.

DISEASE.	INCUBATION.	PERIOD OF INFECTION.
Chicken pox - -	14 days	3 weeks
Measles - - -	12 ,,	4 ,,
German Measles -	18 ,,	3 ,,
Scarlet Fever - .	2 to 7 days	6 to 8 weeks
Whooping Cough -	10 to 14 ,,	6 to 8 ,,
Mumps - - -	21 ,,	3 ,,

Chicken-pox, sometimes called glass-pox, is usually a very mild disorder. The child becomes a little out of sorts and feverish, and in about twenty-four hours is covered with a rash. This appears, at first, in the form of small, red, raised spots, which during the day become filled with a clear watery fluid. The spots do not come out all at once, but in crops ; they are usually specially abundant on the face and back, and about the head : they increase in size, their contents become milky, and they then either burst or dry up, forming small scabs which, about the end of a week, fall off, leaving red stains upon the skin, which slowly disappear. In some cases, especially if irritated, a spot may leave a scar.

The child will probably require no medicine at all, but must be kept indoors whilst it has the rash, and should be kept from scratching the spots, especially those on the face. The bowels should be regulated if necessary. The period of infection lasts about a fortnight, but is not over until every scab has fallen off.

Measles is very infectious, even before the appearance of the rash, so that though a child may be separated from his companions on the first appearance of the rash, the others are almost certain to contract the disease.

At first the child becomes dull, heavy, and feverish, and appears utterly miserable. Sneezing, and running at the eyes and nose set in, and usually a hacking dry cough makes its appearance. In young children there may be convulsions. On the fourth day of illness the rash comes out, first on the face and behind the ears, and then spreading to the arms, belly, and legs. The mucous membrane of the mouth and throat are also generally affected, so that the child will often complain of a sore throat. The rash first appears in the form of small red pimples, which quickly increase in size and run together, forming irregular blotches. Whilst the eruption is at its height, the face appears bloated and swollen, and the hands tight and bursting. At this time it is quite common for the temperature to be about 105°, and accompanied by delirium, but as soon as the rash begins to fade, *i.e.*, about the sixth or seventh day of the disease, the fever suddenly drops and the child becomes convalescent. The eruption fades in the same order that it appeared.

While the rash is out the child must be kept strictly in bed, unless indeed it be very young, when it may be nursed. Great care must be taken lest it catch cold, and for this reason it is best to let it wear a flannel night-gown with long sleeves.

The most troublesome part of the complaint is usually the cough. If the throat be sore, give thick barley-water ; black currant tea should be given sparingly, as diarrhœa may set in, which is difficult to control. During the fever stage the child will probably suffer from inflamed eyes ; they should be bathed with warm water, and the room kept darkened. About the twelfth day the skin often scales in little flakes. In cases in which the rash does not come out well, the child may become very ill and convulsions set in ; a hot bath is then called for.

Some epidemics of measles seem to take a malignant form, but as a rule, with care, children do well.

There is a popular idea that healthy children should be allowed to mix with those who have contracted the disease, so that they may get it over early and have done with it. The idea is not a good one. The disease is not such a trivial affair as many imagine, and many a mother has had to regret that she did not take more care of her children in isolating the sick one from the very beginning.

The period of infection lasts a month from the commencement of the attack. Of course, all the usual rules of disinfection must be carried out before the child be pronounced clean.

If the fever keep up, and the child be ill after the rash have disappeared, some complication must be feared. The commonest dangerous complications are bronchitis or inflammation of the lungs, but an attack of measles is liable to be followed by various evil consequences :—

(1). A chronic state of low health, which should be treated with tonics, and change to the sea.

(2). Bronchitis, inflammation of the lungs, or consumption.

(3). Inflammation of the eyes.

(4). Inflammation of the ears.

German measles is a disease quite distinct from ordinary measles, and an attack of the one will not afford any protection from the other. As a rule the disease is milder than true measles. The rash appears on the second day of the illness, and is usually very irritable ; the glands down the side of the neck are generally enlarged and somewhat painful; cough is usually absent; convalescence is rapid, and is sometimes accompanied by peeling.

Scarlet fever or *Scarlatina.*—Vomiting or convulsions may be the first symptoms. The *throat* is almost always affected, being very red and swollen; the glands in the neck often swell and become tender. The skin feels very hot and burning, and the rash comes out on the second day. The eruption shows itself at first as small red spots, which quickly spread until the whole skin presents a scarlet appearance, with the original spots showing through, so that the child looks like a boiled lobster sprinkled with cayenne pepper. There is no disease so unequal in its attacks as scarlet fever; usually infants do very well.

After the rash has reached its height the fever slowly abates, and in a week should have entirely disappeared. Peeling of the skin generally begins about the eighth day, the size of the flakes depending upon the thickness of the skin. It is often not completed under six weeks from its commencement. Infection is very liable to hang about in the clothes of the patient, or in the paper on the walls of the room, and is at its height during the peeling stage, so that the child must be kept strictly isolated until that be quite over. In a mild case the child may be almost well at the end of a fortnight, and, if desired, can be sent to the Mary Wardell Scarlet Fever Convalescent Home, Stanmore, Middlesex, where it can have fresh air and exercise combined with skilled supervision.

The chief complications are :—

(1). Inflammation of the kidneys and dropsy. This usually takes place during the peeling stage, and may have been caused by a chill.

(2.) Rheumatism. . This is dangerous on account of the damage that may be done to the heart.

(3). Inflammation of the eye or ear.

Like typhoid fever, scarlet fever may be spread by means of contaminated milk, and is an additional reason why all milk should be boiled, so that any germs which are present may be destroyed.

Small-pox.—This disease is practically quite unknown in infants that have been efficiently vaccinated. The rash appears on the third day, and the eyes are specially liable to suffer.

The younger the child, the more likely is the disease to prove fatal. During an epidemic of small pox, infants should be vaccinated when a few days old.

Typhoid fever is rare in infants. It is characterized by diarrhœa and fever. A few spots generally make their appearance on the abdomen about the tenth day of illness. No solid food *of any description* should be given, as the fever is one in which inflammation of the bowels is always present, and any irritation to them in the way of solid food or fruit may cause sudden death.

Whooping Cough.—This disease is very contagious. It begins with an ordinary cough, which may last some weeks before the characteristic " whoop " makes its appearance. The infection of the disease lasts about six weeks, but the risk of infection cannot be said to be positively over until the child quite ceases whooping. In bad cases the fits of coughing will come on every half-hour, or even oftener, and are often accompanied by vomiting. Owing to the violence of the cough, bleeding may occur from the nose, or, more rarely, from the ears, and hæmorrhage beneath the mucous membrane of the eyes is very common. If the child have any bronchitis, bed is the best place for it, and a steam kettle with carbolic lotion may be used in the room.

In ordinary cases it is best to have a day and a night room. Early in the day, burn sulphur in the night room, leave the windows open all the afternoon, have a fire, and let the child sleep there. In this way the attack will probably be much shortened. A lamp burning cresoline (to be had of any chemist) may be used in the day room.

If the chest be very stuffy, it may be well rubbed, in front of the fire, with some embrocation. If the child vomit during the fit of coughing, light food, *e.g.*, milk and water or raw beef juice, should be given directly after the attack. The duration of the disease is very variable. The chief dangers are bronchitis, inflammation of the lungs, and consumption. If the patient be rickety, the dangers of whooping cough are greatly increased. When the disease passes into a chronic stage, *i.e.*, after about two or three weeks, in suitable weather the child should be out as much as possible, and later on a change to the seaside will often effect wonders.

The child while still whooping should not be allowed to go near other children ; and it should be remembered that the contagion can be transmitted by the mother or nurse.

Diphtheria.—This is a contagious disease characterized by the deposit of a whitish-grey membrane, which usually appears in the throat. There is fever, loss of appetite, lassitude, and a difficulty of swallowing. Sometimes, however, these symptoms are so slight as not to be noticed at all. On examining the throat the diphtheritic membrane is usually plainly to be seen on the tonsils, uvula, or adjacent parts. Vomiting is often present. Hoarseness or loss of voice points to a spread of the membrane to the windpipe : a copious discharge from the nose may indicate a spread of the disease to that organ. Lumps, due to enlarged glands, usually appear on each side of the jaw.

A doctor should always be sent for *at once*. A case of diphtheria, however mild it may appear to be at first, may prove fatal in the long run. When the child is first taken ill, it is not always possible to say whether the disease will turn out to be diphtheria or not, but it is best to isolate the patient and put him to bed at once.

In cases where the mother decides to look after the child, she must be completely shut off from her other children.

During the first few days the child will probably have great difficulty in swallowing, and will keep its mouth open, allowing the saliva to trickle on to the pillow. The great thing is to keep the strength up as much as possible. Stimulants will probably be necessary, and food in the form of milk, eggs, soups, beef-tea, etc., given in small quantities very frequently. In bad cases the child must be kept perfectly quiet, and not even allowed to sit up in bed to take its food. The three chief dangers are—

(1). *Exhaustion.* In some cases, though the throat itself goes on well, the complexion will get of a waxy hue, the pulse becomes slower and slower, and the child will gradually pass away. Sometimes, when the child has been allowed to make some sudden movement, or has suddenly sat up in bed, it has dropped back dead. Vomiting occurring after the first few days is a very bad sign, and quickly leads to exhaustion.

(2). *Suffocation.* If the membrane spread to the windpipe, the breathing will become laboured, the nostrils will dilate, and the ribs fall in at each inspiration, and unless something be done, the child will die suffocated. In suitable cases, opening the windpipe affords the only hope. The operation itself is not a dangerous one, and the longer it is deferred, the less likely is it to prove successful.

(3). *Paralysis.* If, when the child swallows, some of the fluid returns through its nose, some paralysis of the soft palate may be suspected. Squint, or weakness of a limb, are also signs of paralysis. Sometimes the paralysis spreads until the child cannot move at all, and it may prove fatal; but, as a rule, it is quite recovered from. No case is hopeless.

All orders from the doctor should be carefully carried out. Sometimes the throat has to be sprayed or painted every two or three hours, and the mother should be very careful while doing so, that the child do not spit or cough in her face; indeed, it is best to wear a small mask over the face for protection. Nearly all cases are now treated by the injection of anti-diphtheritic serum, which has very greatly reduced the mortality of this terrible disease.

Bad drains and contaminated milk are the two great causes of diphtheria, and should both be carefully considered in trying to discover the origin of the disease.

It is astonishing how long the infection lasts, and careful disinfection must be carried out.

The diseases which are most likely to be confounded with diphtheria are quinsy and scarlet fever.

CROUP AND CHILD CROWING.

The common history of an attack of croup is as follows :—the child, apparently in the midst of good health, suddenly wakens up in the early hours of the morning, gasping for breath. Its face is blue and covered with a cold perspiration, and the breathing is slow, laboured, and noisy. The voice is reduced to a whisper, and there is an occasional harsh cough. After a time, varying from half an hour to an hour, the symptoms slowly subside, and the child falls asleep, to wake in the morning quite well, with the exception of a slight hoarseness, and an occasional cough. The child is very liable to get another attack on the following night, about the same hour. Although very alarming, these attacks are very seldom fatal. The child, for the time, seems on the eve of suffocation, but, as a matter of fact, there is not very much danger. The quickest way to cut short an attack is to make the child vomit. For this purpose give a teaspoonful of ipecacuanha wine, and repeat it if necessary. A hot bath with a tablespoonful of mustard in it, will also prove beneficial.

The commonest exciting factor in this disease seems to be exposure to damp cold.

Laryngismus stridulus, or *Child Crowing*.—This disease is characterized by the child being suddenly seized with a spasm of its breath. The child stops breathing, turns blue, clenches its hands, and then suddenly draws in its breath, with a low crow, and is well again. In those who are subject to this complaint any sudden shock will produce an attack, *e.g.*, tossing the child up in the air, or giving it a smack. The voice remains unaffected. The attacks are very frightening, and are sometimes, though rarely, fatal. Should a seizure seem to last longer than usual, dash cold water in the child's face, or give it sharp smacks on the back. It is a disease that children grow out of as they get older. A doctor will probably order bromide of ammonium, which will assist in the recovery.

The general treatment is that of rickets ; nearly all children subject to child-crowing are, at the same time, rickety. Feed the child properly, give it plenty of air and sunlight, and the fits will probably soon cease for ever.

RICKETS.

This common disease among children may almost be defined as " wry bones," for though it is not confined to them, it is principally to be seen in the bones. Rickets is a disease affecting the whole body, although it is not usually recognized by mothers until the changes in the bones are noticeable. The ends of the long bones enlarge, and produce swellings at the ankles and wrists. Little lumps also often form where the ribs join the breast bone in front, and the chest becomes triangular shaped, like that of a pigeon. As soon as any pressure is brought to bear upon the bones they bend ; *e.g.*, as soon as the child begins to walk, and the weight of the body has to be borne by the legs, they will give, producing what is called " bow-legs." If the child sits up much the back will bend. The bones being so soft are very liable to fracture (*vide* " green-stick " fracture p. 106). The head enlarges, and the anterior fontanelle does not properly close. The teeth are late in coming.

One of the earliest symptoms of the disease is profuse *sweating* of the head and neck, especially during sleep, and the child will often throw off the bedclothes and lie naked, even in winter. The belly gets big and protuberant, and the motions are often offensive. Although very likely the child does not seem to lose flesh, it will get flabby and will not like to be touched, as it becomes tender all over. If the child have begun to walk it will become unsteady, and the enlargement and bending of the bones will soon be noticed. A rickety child is very liable to attacks of bronchitis, croup, diarrhœa, etc. It is very important that mothers and nurses should be able to detect the earliest symptoms of rickets. A doctor is often consulted for the croup or bronchitis, which might have been entirely averted if the true cause had been earlier recognized. A cold which a healthy child would throw off in a few days, will often in a rickety one develop into bronchitis, and may even end fatally. The nervous system of rickety children is very easily upset, so that convulsions and child-crowing are common.

Rickets *is a preventable disease*, and ought never to occur in the children of mothers who have read this little book. The causes are bad food, bad air, damp, cold rooms, want of sunlight, want of exercise, and want of cleanliness.

To prevent rickets children must be—

(1). Fed on food suitable to their age.

(2). Kept in well ventilated, dry rooms, free from bad smells.

(3). Given plenty of light and sun-baths.

(4). Given out-door exercise every fine day, and indoor exercise every wet day.

(5). Given soap and water baths at least once a day.

Now these are not impossible rules, except perhaps to a very few, and even then a little ingenuity will often accomplish wonders.

Each rule has been carefully considered in its practical aspect in other parts of the book, and it is to be hoped that every mother will try to work out and improve upon the various suggestions made.

Supposing, however, that all the five rules have apparently been faithfully carried out, and yet the first symptoms of rickets appear, what is the cause ? In all probability the first rule has been *unwittingly* broken, *e.g.*, in the case of a child with a weak digestion, the milk has been diluted to such an extent that the child has been half starved. The great remedies here will be *raw meat juice* and *cream* or *cod-liver oil*.

If a child with commencing rickets has reached the age of crawling or walking, its legs must be bound together during the day with a piece of flannel. At night leave the legs loose, so that it may kick about as much as it likes. The only use of having the legs bound together is to prevent the child standing or crawling, because it must be remembered that, directly weight is put upon the bones they will bend.

Bad cases of rickets may require splints, but if the child be kept off its feet from the very beginning, and the five rules above given be carefully attended to, it will quickly recover and the bones get strong.

Rickety infants are liable to an acid form of indigestion, and bear starchy foods badly ; what they require are eggs, milk, raw meat juice, and cream. Kepler's extract of malt makes a capital aid to their digestion, and cod-liver oil is generally the only medicine called for. With young infants a tablespoonful of saccharated lime water in each bottle, replacing the same amount of barley water, is often beneficial. Rickets, although not a fatal disease in itself, may, indirectly, cause death from bronchitis or diarrhœa.

It is interesting to know that formerly it was found impossible to rear young lions at the Zoological Gardens, as they always succumbed to rickets. Now that raw meat, pounded bones, and cod-liver oil have been added to their diet, the cubs have been brought up without any difficulty.

SKIN AFFECTIONS.

If there be one thing more than another upon which a mother is apt to pride herself, it is the fact that her baby always has such a clear skin. Any skin disease, however slight, thus becomes a source of great annoyance, not only to the child but also to the mother. The skin of a child is very delicate and sensitive, and any chafing or irritation, *e.g.*, the using of a coarse soap, will probably bring out a rash.

Nævus, or *Mother's Mark*, is a very common congenital skin affection, which may occur anywhere, and consists of dilated blood-vessels, which may be either of a bright scarlet or dark purple colour ; the blood can generally be pressed out, so that the spot becomes quite pale.

It really exists at birth, though it may not be noticed for some time later. If situated on a part that does not show, it had better be left alone, providing it is not increasing in size. One that has remained unchanged for a long time, may suddenly increase in size, and then something will have to be done. Different nævi require different treatment ; cures are usually effected by painting them with acids, vaccinating them, and tying them, or, in some cases cutting them out. Some nævi are specially adapted for treatment by electricity.

Red Gum.—This rash usually shows itself in infants under a year old, in the form of small, bright, red spots, generally on the face, but often covering the whole chest and body. As a rule the rash is not very irritable, and begins to disappear in a few days. Fresh crops of spots are, however, very apt to come out. The appearance of red gum usually indicates some amount of indigestion and acidity, and is often associated with teething. The best thing is to give a dose of magnesia to clear the bowels, and five grains of bi-carbonate of soda, about as much as will lie on a sixpenny bit, in a little milk to correct the acidity. The rash may be dusted with starch powder.

Eczema.—This eruption has the appearance of a bright, red, moist surface covered with dried-up discharge in the form of crusts or scabs. The most common parts to be affected are the face and scalp and behind the ears ; the groins and insides of the joints are also very liable to be attacked. In some instances a child is one mass of eczema from head to foot. In cases of acute eczema, the irritation is very great, and if allowed, the child will almost tear himself to pieces. The discharge from the sores, if allowed to run over the healthy skin, will irritate it, and cause the disease to spread.

In treatment the great thing is to find out the cause, which is commonly some error in diet, *e.g.*, bringing up a young infant on starch food, which causes irritation of the bowels, indigestion, and irritation of the skin. Any irritation, *e.g.*, that of friction or rubbing of the part, that set up by lice, or that of teething, may very quickly induce an attack of eczema. Scrofulous children are also very subject to this disease.

All sources of irritation should be removed, and, if necessary, the child must wear gloves at night to prevent him scratching himself.

Soap should not be employed for washing the part, but oatmeal water or sweet oil may be used when cleansing is absolutely necessary, though the less it be washed the better. The ordinary soaps contain free soda and potash, and these act very injuriously in eczema.

Sea air is bad for eczema, as it contains so much salt.

The bowels must be regulated and the food carefully attended to. In older children sweets, raw fruit, and much meat act injuriously.

Locally, the places may be gently sponged with a solution of bi-carbonate of soda, containing oxide of zinc, or a solution known as Startin's paint. Lotions are most useful during the discharging stage of the disease, and ointments during the scaly stage. It is of no use to apply any medicament on the top of a lot of scabs. The part should first be well soaked in oil, and the crusts picked off ; if, however, they still adhere, a poultice had better be used. The best ointments are the zinc, and the white precipitate, which last should be used diluted with lard.

The general health is of great importance, and Kepler's extract of malt, steel wine, or cod-liver oil should be given when required.

Eczema is often a very difficult thing to get rid of, and relapses are common. After the child seems quite well again, any little irritation, *e.g.*, the east wind, will very likely bring back the disease as bad as ever.

Nettle Rash or Urticaria.—An acute attack of nettle rash is usually due to some error in diet, the rash appearing as raised white lumps surrounded by a halo of congestion. The irritation is intense, and may be accompanied by diarrhœa and vomiting.

The best treatment is to give a dose of castor oil, and a bath containing two ounces of soda to three gallons of warm water, and, after drying, to dust on some oxide of zinc powder. The attack usually lasts two or three days. Sometimes, however, a chronic form attacks children, lasting in some cases months or even years, getting better at times and then breaking out again as badly as ever. The treatment is most disheartening, but attention must be paid to the bowels and diet. Sulphur, given internally, often does good. The itching may be allayed by a lotion of Liquor Carbonis Detergens, a tablespoonful to a pint of water, dabbed on with a sponge.

Ringworm.—This complaint is caused, not by a worm, but by a vegetable fungus. It is very contagious, and spreads by children using the same towels and brushes, putting on each other's caps, or by direct contact during play or sleep. The eruption is somewhat irritable, and often causes scratching. At first it appears as a dull red circular patch, often covered with little scales ; this patch slowly increases in size, fading somewhat in the centre as it spreads.

If ringworm attack the head, the hairs in the affected part will break off near the surface of the skin, leaving a bald patch. The hairs do not drop out by the roots, but snap off, so that a small portion appears above the skin. These broken-off hairs are very characteristic of the disease, and at once distinguish it from patches of mere local baldness.

The treatment is to be directed to killing the fungus, which is the real cause of the disease. A patch of ringworm on the arm or leg is very easily cured, but ringworm of the scalp is a most tiresome and vexatious thing ; month after month the mother may diligently persevere in the treatment, and yet the case may remain uncured.

If ringworm attack the scalp, and there be several distinct patches, it will be quicker in the end to have the head completely shaved, and to let the child wear a skull cap. Before applying any remedy, the patch should be cleansed with hot water and soap. An ointment of a drachm of salicylic acid to an ounce of vaseline, thoroughly rubbed in, is often used. Iodine in the form of the liniment, or in the case of young children the tincture, may be painted on. Another good lotion is sulphurous acid, rubbed in with a rag ; its smell is, however, rather objectionable. Stronger remedies may sometimes be required.

The child must have a separate brush and towel, and of course must be kept away from school until quite well.

In some cases, the pulling out of diseased hairs by forceps will hasten the cure. It is always difficult, and often indeed impossible, for a mother to know when the disease is really cured, but a doctor can always tell by means of the microscope if there be any fungus still left.

The Itch, or *Scabies*, is a skin eruption, dependent upon the irritation of an insect, the itch insect, in the skin. The parts mostly affected are the hands, feet, and buttocks. The irritation is always great, and the scratching of the infant is liable to set up eczema. At first the eruption appears as little watery heads, which are soon filled with matter.

The female insects burrow in the skin, whilst the male crawl about the skin and clothes. They are very small, not being as large as a pin's head. The face is never attacked.

The treatment is as follows :—Give the child a hot bath, using coal tar soap, and being especially vigorous over the affected parts. Keep the child in the water about a quarter of an hour, so that the skin may become thoroughly softened ; next dry, and well rub in a mixture of a teaspoonful of balsam of Peru to one ounce of vaseline. All the clothes should be baked in the oven. Balsam of Peru is better to use than sulphur, being less irritating. Put the child to bed, and in the morning give a warm bath to get rid of the ointment. Of course the itch is very catching, and the mother and nurse are very liable to take it from the child.

Lice.—These disgusting insects, politely called pediculi by the doctor, cause very great irritation of the part affected. Their favourable point of attack is the head, and, by diligent search, they can be easily discovered when present. The eggs are of an oval shape and are glued on to the hairs. Lice cause eczema, especially that form which is situated at the back of the neck, and the glands in the neighbourhood are often enlarged.

The usual treatment is to wash the head with a carbolic acid or sulphurous acid lotion, and use the staves-acre ointment. The strength of the lotion should be one part of acid to fifty of water, and care must be taken

that it does not run down the face or into the eyes.
Washing the head with corrosive sublimate soap is also
very efficacious, while methylated spirit applied with a
sponge will detach the nits from the hairs.

WORMS.

There are three varieties of worms by which a child
may be infested : the tape worm, round worm, and
thread worm. The symptoms that may be caused by
worms are :—Irritation and consequent scratching at
the anus, grinding of the teeth, picking at the nose, disturbance of the bowels, and capricious appetite. In
many cases, however, the presence of worms gives rise to
no symptoms at all.

Tape Worm.—It is rare for tapeworm to infest infants.
By appropriate means they can pretty easily be got
rid of. Flat pieces of the worm are passed with the
motions of the child. A cure will not take place until
the head of the animal be passed.

Round Worms are several inches long, and have somewhat the appearance of a common earth worm. They
vary in number, but are usually single. It is not a very
uncommon thing for the child to expel the worm from its
mouth by vomiting. The usual treatment is santonin,
given under a doctor's orders : it may be mixed with a
little powdered sugar, and given at bed-time. A dose of
castor oil is generally given the next morning. In two
or three days' time the treatment may have to be
repeated.

Thread Worms.—These worms, when present, usually
exist in large numbers. They are only about a quarter
of an inch long, and inhabit the lower bowel, and often
escape from the anus and crawl about in its vicinity. If
there be much mucus secreted from the bowel, it seems
to afford a convenient resting place for the worms to
breed and multiply.

The best treatment is injections into the lower bowel
of salt and water, a teaspoonful to a pint, or an infusion
of quassia of the same strength. In young children,
not more than three or four ounces of injection should
be used at a time. It is well to repeat the operation

for a few days, night and morning, at the same time keeping the bowels open.

In some cases it is best not to give injections, but to give santonin, the same as for round worms. Worm cakes are sold by chemists, but, as a rule, are not very satisfactory, the quantity of santonin they contain being very uncertain.

In all cases of suspected worms the motions should be carefully examined, as it is impossible to arrive at a correct diagnosis unless the worms, or their eggs be seen.

DIARRHŒA.

Of all diseases to which infants are subject, summer diarrhœa is by far the most fatal. Of 15,000 deaths among children in New York, 13,000 were from this complaint. In olden times, at the Foundling Hospitals, of every 100 infants brought up by hand, 60 to 80 died of diarrhœa before they were a year old.

The bowels of a healthy infant usually act two or three times a day at the commencement of its career, the motions being of a bright yellow colour, not markedly offensive, and containing but few traces of undigested casein. If a child be passing six or seven motions daily, it is probably passing, at the same time, a good deal of undigested food, in the form of large white masses of casein.

The great causes of infantile diarrhœa are errors in diet and want of cleanliness.

The mucous membrane of the child's stomach is exceedingly delicate, and it is not slow to resent any irritation of its walls. Big curds of solid casein, waltzing round the stomach, are sure to do mischief, and sooner or later will set up vomiting and diarrhœa.

The great preventives are proper food and cleanliness. Any error in diet is liable to cause irritation, and the stomach and intestines are both bent upon getting rid of the offending substance as quickly as possible ; it is no marvel, therefore, that vomiting and diarrhœa often accompany one another. But it is much easier to start a diarrhœa than to stop one.

In an analysis of 710 cases of fatal infantile diarrhœa,

it was found that 393 had had no breast milk, 287 had
been fed on a mixed diet, and that only 30 had been
brought up on breast milk alone.

Infantile diarrhœa is far commoner in summer than in
winter, on account of the greater liability of the food to
ferment and decompose. Sometimes it sets in as a
regular epidemic ; the worst months are June to August.
Hand-fed infants, among the poor, are heavily handi-
capped during the summer months ; it is so easy to
forget that the least trace of sour food will poison a
whole meal, and perhaps endanger the child's life. In
cases where the mother goes out to work, and the infant
is hired out to ignorant people to feed, the mortality
during the summer months is so great that these said
nurses are known as " angel-mongers."

Infantile diarrhœa, or gastro-enteritis, begins by the
bowels acting more frequently than they should do, then
the yellow motions change to a green substance like
chopped spinach, and at last they resemble offensive
ditch water. Their frequency varies very much,
amounting in some cases to three or four times in the
hour. Vomiting is usually set up at the same time.
The rapidity with which infants succumb to this disease
is awful. The breathing becomes quick and shallow,
the anterior fontanelle sinks in, and the child, who at
first was hot and feverish, now lies on its back, collapsed
and cold to the touch. A plump, healthy child may
be almost unrecognizable at the end of three days' time,
the sunken eyes and leaden face giving it quite a different
appearance.

Treatment.—Call in a doctor at once, before the child
becomes hopelessly ill. A diarrhœa should never go on
unchecked. Give the child plenty of air, putting it into
a large cool room. If possible, arrange that different
persons should feed and change the child. Auto-
infection has been proved to play an important part in
the relapses which are so frequent, and therefore the
hands of the one feeding the child should not run any
risk of being contaminated by fæcal discharge. Not
only should soiled napkins be removed immediately,
but the child should be changed in another room to the

one it generally occupies. It should be kept very quiet, lying in a cot near a widely open window, which should be on the cool side of the house in summer. A woollen binder must be worn, and a hot bottle kept near the feet, if they are chilly. Moving from town into the country often proves beneficial.

To persistently give the child food when it is vomiting and has diarrhœa, is absurd, although the mother gives it with the idea of "keeping up the child's strength." The child's inside wants a rest : to feed it up is to take away, may be, its only chance. In bad cases discontinue all milk food. Beat up the whites of two eggs with half-a-pint of thin barley water, and of this give one table-spoonful every hour for twenty-four hours—or longer. Should the child be collapsed, brandy, in the proportions before given, can be added to the mixture every third or fourth hour, and a warm bath with a small tablespoonful of mustard in it will help to revive the infant. Some-times two teaspoonfuls of raw meat juice may be alternated with the egg mixture with great advantage. Whey may also be given for the same length of time. After twenty-four hours in mild cases, or forty-eight in more severe ones, milk which has been fully peptonized should be cautiously begun in small doses, returning very gradually to the usual diet. To sum up the treatment :—Strict attention to diet, plenty of fresh air and scrupulous cleanliness.

Dysentery.—Dysenteric diarrhœa is characterized by a discharge of blood and mucus from the bowel. This disease is not, as a rule, due to errors in diet, but to a chill of the bowels, setting up inflammation. Usually, there is a good deal of straining and bearing down of the bowel, and at the outset there may be fever and vomiting.

The great preventive of dysentery is the proper protection of the bowels from cold; for this reason a stomach belt should be worn by day and night (*vide* pages 8 and 9). The line of treatment is to give the bowels as much rest as possible, allowing only barley water and egg as before described.

If a child pass blood and mucus with great straining,

and at the same time have constipation, a doctor should be sent for at once, as the child probably has *intussusception of the bowel, i.e.,* one portion of the bowel has slipped into another like an inverted finger of a glove. Any purgative will make matters much worse, and an early operation is generally required to save life.

JAUNDICE.

It is a very common thing for a child of three days old to become jaundiced and yellow all over. This, however, is of no consequence, and disappears in a week or so. In older children, jaundice is usually due to a cold on the liver, which produces congestion of that organ, and a temporary stoppage of the bile ducts. The urine is of a dark yellow colour, and stains the napkins. The motions are of a pale white colour, showing an absence of bile. Sickness may be present, and the bowels are generally confined. The stomach should be kept warm, and well covered up, and, unless the weather be warm, the child should be kept strictly indoors until the jaundice has quite disappeared. The disease requires careful management, but need cause no anxiety.

SCROFULA, STRUMA, OR KING'S EVIL.

This disease has been called the scourge of England. It is hereditary, and should two scrofulous persons marry, their children will almost certainly become affected sooner or later.

Scrofula manifests itself in many ways, notably in diseases of the glands and joints, and in older persons in disease of the lungs, causing consumption.

A child who inherits a scrofulous constitution will require very great care from the time of its birth. A slight illness which in a healthy child is quickly recovered from, will often, in the scrofulous child, lay the seeds of a fatal disease; *e.g.*, a diarrhœa set up by improper feeding may prove the starting point of consumption of the bowels.

If a child has a marked scrofulous tendency, it will probably carry it all through life, but if there be only a slight tendency, it may be eradicated by careful hygienic treatment. The successful treatment of scrofula does not lie in medicines, but in suitable food in sufficient quantity, plenty of outdoor exercise, thorough ventilation of all the rooms, supplemented by country or sea air as often as possible. In weaned children, a large quantity of milk should still be systematically given. The appetite of scrofulous children is often very capricious, but a good allowance of milk, milk puddings, eggs, etc., should be firmly insisted upon. To give way to a child's whims in these matters often means the first step in a downward course of health, and the great majority of children, both in wealthy and poor households, are underfed in these requisite articles of diet.

Cod-liver oil, either as an emulsion or in malt, is most valuable in these cases, and should regularly be given through the winter months, when it is increasingly important to keep up the supply of animal fat.

Scrofulous children are very liable to swollen glands in the neck ; these will often require removal, as, if allowed to burst, they may go on discharging for many months, and leave very ugly scars. Discharge from the ears, which is also very common in these cases, should never be neglected, as total deafness may result. A swelling of the stomach, accompanied by great wasting of the child, is usually a sign of consumption of the bowels. The eyes and eyelids are very liable to suffer, and will require special care. Convulsions, squint, screaming, with rolling of the head from side to side, are signs of a scrofulous inflammation of the brain. Scrofulous disease of the joints is described elsewhere.

Enough has been said to show parents the necessity for a watchful care and special supervision, if there be reason to suspect a scrofulous taint in their family.

Strumous children being generally " delicate," it is often considered necessary that they should be coddled and shut up nearly all the winter in hot ill-ventilated rooms. If the child really be scrofulous, and be treated in this way, it will afford a splendid opportunity for the scrofula to develop and rapidly increase. Always bear in mind that they require *more* air than other children, and if they be warmly clothed and accustomed to it, cold air will not hurt them, but will act as a tonic. If obliged to be kept in for wet weather, the regular ventilation of the rooms should be supervised by the mother herself.

Usually, nothing picks up a strumous child like going to the seaside, especially the east coast.

SCURVY.

The now very general use of peptonized and sterilized milk and patent foods has caused the disease known as infantile scurvy to be far more common than formerly, and in contradistinction to rickets, it is found more amongst the well-to-do than the poor.

It is characterized by tender bones, swellings on the limbs, hæmorrhages under the skin, spongy gums, anæmia, earthy complexion and smell, and great debility, and is caused by the lack of *fresh food*. It is most common between the ages of six and eighteen months; and its occurrence calls for an immediate change to fresh boiled milk, raw meat juice, and mashed potato, but of course medical advice must be sought.

HIP DISEASE.

This very rarely attacks infants ; indeed, it is very rare under three years old, but its early recognition is so important that a few words are necessary. To take it in time is the great thing. A child, generally between four and ten years old, will begin to cry out in its sleep ; it is a sudden, sharp cry, not necessarily waking the child. Soon the child will be noticed to walk with a slight limp, and complain of pain, probably in one knee ; he does not jump about and play as usual, but goes carefully, as if he were afraid of any sudden jar to the foot. He should be taken to a doctor at once. The disease is a scrofulous inflammation of the joint, and the treatment will require great patience.

Complete rest to the joint is required, and in order to carry this out, the child will probably have to lie on his back, quite flat, for several months, and have a weight attached to the bad leg.

If all goes well, after some months he will be allowed to get up and walk on crutches, having the hip fixed in a splint.

In bad cases, abscesses form round the joint, and an operation may be necessary. Even in favourable cases there may be a perceptible limp in the walk after the child gets quite well.

Hip disease is very serious, not only with regard to the joint, but even the life of the child. Poor persons had far better, if possible, get the child into a hospital ; the case will be one certainly of months, possibly of years.

A table, with specially arranged apparatus, has been invented to enable a child to play with his toys whilst lying on his back.

AILMENTS OF THE EYES.

Ophthalmia is an inflammation of the membrane covering the eyeball and lids. We have already seen how prone new-born infants are to suffer from this disease. Unfortunately, ophthalmia is very common in older children, especially those who are strumous.

The white of the eye becomes red and swollen, and a thick yellow discharge exudes from it. In some cases the swelling is so great that the child cannot open the lid. The lids are generally glued together in the morning by the discharge which has been secreted during the night.

The great cause of ophthalmia is overcrowding and want of fresh air. In every case of eye trouble a doctor must be consulted at once, as delay may prove dangerous. The discharge is very contagious, and one eye will often infect the other. The child must be kept separate, and every precaution be taken to prevent the disease spreading to others. The eye should be cleansed and bathed with warm water and absorbent wool, a fresh piece being used each time, after which an astringent lotion of alum, sulphate of zinc, or nitrate of silver, half a grain or one grain to the ounce, is often employed. The lotion must really get inside the eye or it will do no good. The child should be taken on one's lap, the head

thrown well back, and the lids gently separated. A
pipette with a little india-rubber cap, sold for the
purpose, is the best instrument to use for dropping
in the lotion. In bad cases this operation may require
repeating every hour the child is awake. The lids
should be smeared with a little vaseline to prevent
their sticking. The general health must not be forgotten, and an abundance of fresh air is absolutely
necessary. If ophthalmia be neglected, the inflammation
may spread to the ball of the eye itself and destroy
sight.

There is a form of ophthalmia which affects the part
covering the inner surface of the eyelids, which is apt to
assume a chronic form, and gives rise to what are called
granular lids. In this form of the disease, the constant
movement of the lid keeps up the irritation, and the
affection becomes troublesome. In many of these cases
the lids will require turning inside out and touching with
a stick of blue-stone daily.

Ulcer on the Eye.—An ulcer on the front part of the
eye or cornea is always accompanied by pain, watering
of the eye, and a fear of light. It always denotes ill
health or scrofula, and may follow an attack of measles
or scarlet fever. The eye generally waters a good deal,
and the child will absolutely refuse to allow it to be
looked at. The general treatment consists of tonics,
e.g., cod-liver oil, steel wine, or Kepler's malt extract,
good food and plenty of fresh air. The eye should be
carefully protected by a shade or veil whilst the child
is out-of-doors, but whilst in-doors it is better to slightly
darken the room. To keep the child shut up in a dark
room from morning till night to mope and fret will
prove most disastrous.

The child must be taken to a doctor, who will probably
order an atropine lotion to be dropped into the eye twice
a day, and perhaps a blister on the temple.

An ulcer on the cornea, even when healed, leaves
a little white spot or scar behind it, which, if over
the pupil, may interfere with the sight. Neglected
cases of corneal ulcer may lead to the destruction of
the eyeball.

Inflammation of Eyelashes.—Among poor children an inflammation of the roots of the eyelashes is a very common disorder. The edges of the lids become red and irritable, and a thick secretion is poured out which glues the lids together. Scabs form and the lashes drop out, forming a very unpleasant spectacle. The great line of treatment is cleanliness and tonics. The scabs should be bathed off, and a little dilute yellow oxide of mercury ointment smeared on. A child that has once had the disease is very liable to have it again.

Squint.—Cases of squint or cross eyes are usually due to some slight malformation of the eyeball, and should be seen by a doctor at once. Some cases can be cured by spectacles, others require an operation.

Headaches over the forehead, and blurring of objects, point to a defect in vision, and the child had better be examined at once, as it may be ruining its sight.

THE EAR.

Otitis, or inflammation of the middle ear, is very painful, and reveals itself by bad ear-ache. There will probably be persistent crying, rolling of the head from side to side, fever, and loss of appetite, and a tenderness just behind the ear. At this stage, hot fomentations and poultices may give relief. The doctor, who should always be sent for at once, will probably give a purge and perhaps order a leech. Otitis generally goes on to the formation of matter. This matter, being unable to get out, causes great pain, but in time it usually penetrates the drum of the ear, and appears outside as a thick yellow discharge, often smelling very offensively. As soon as the matter appears the pain is generally relieved. The surgeon often anticipates the opening of the abscess, and so saves the child a good deal of pain. The ear must now be kept very clean, and gently syringed several times a day with a warm solution of Condy's fluid, after which it is well to gently insert a fresh piece of antiseptic wool.

Otitis is very liable to occur in the course of measles or scarlet fever, or during teething. Discharge from the ear should never be lightly looked upon or neglected.

In spite of all care, deafness may ensue ; and not only so, the inflammation may even spread to the brain, and so cause death.

CONVULSIONS.

These are usually one of the greatest horrors of a young mother. Nothing is more alarming than to see baby, who a few moments ago was looking the picture of health, suddenly turn blue and rigid, all the muscles twitch and become convulsed, the eyes turn up with a fixed unconscious stare, while, to all appearance, in a few more seconds all will be over.

The first thing to do is to loosen the child's clothing, so that there may be nothing tight round the neck, and then to open the mouth by forcing the finger between the gums, so as to allow a free passage of air into the chest. In older children, a spoon or tooth brush can be used instead of the finger. A hot bath may then be given, the head being sponged with cold water at the same time. The usual duration of a fit is about one or two minutes, although they may last much longer. The child may die suffocated during the fit.

The commonest cause of convulsions is an overloaded stomach ; in such cases an emetic is called for. Fits are far more common in rickety children than in healthy ones. Constipation or worms may also excite an attack. Childish ailments, *e.g.*, measles or scarlet fever, are often ushered in by a fit : in some instances it is the first indication of an attack of inflammation of the brain, or of epilepsy. A doctor will usually be able to put his finger at once on the cause of the fit, and so prevent a recurrence.

The so-called *inward convulsions*, in which a young baby has blueness round the mouth and twitchings of the muscles of the face, with half-closed eyes, must not be confounded with true convulsions, but are due to flatulence, and can easily be relieved by a little carbonate of soda in water.

INFANTILE PARALYSIS.

This is a form of paralysis which is fairly common in children under four years old. The legs are usually affected, one or both, though more rarely the upper extremities suffer. The disease may begin with a fit or a feverish attack. In some cases, however, the child may go to bed apparently quite well, and in the morning be found to have complete paralysis of one or both legs. The disease is an inflammation of the spinal cord. The causes are usually stated to be exposure to heat or cold, and over-walking. The paralysed part is quite helpless, but its sensation is perfect. After a few days, it is usual for the paralysis to get a little better, and for some amount of power to return. Wasting of the affected part sets in, so that it becomes much smaller than the other side : it is also cold and bluish. In bad cases the limb is utterly useless. Much can be done by patience and perseverance.

(1). *Clothing :* Always keep the limb warm, day and night. Make the child wear an extra stocking of thick wool, coming well above the knee.

(2). *Rubbing :* this should be done regularly, night and morning, for a quarter of an hour at a time, care being taken to always rub upwards, *i.e.*, towards the body. But besides actual rubbing, the muscles should be kneaded, squeezed, and shampooed. If the expense of a trained masseuse is prohibitive, it will be well for the mother or nurse to take some lessons in massage, in order to carry out this line of treatment.

(3). *Douching :* which should be effected by pouring a large jug of hot water over the limb, followed by a jug of cold water, after which the limb should be rubbed dry with a fairly coarse towel, to produce a glow on the skin. Many use Tidman's sea salt in the water.

(4). *Electricity :* This, after a few lessons, can be applied by the mother at home. An effective Faradic battery can now be bought for about twenty-five shillings. Care should always be taken not to apply the current too strong or for too long a time at one sitting.

Progress will always be slow, and treatment must be carried out systematically, and for a long time. Probably the arm or leg will always be weak, and will get sooner tired than the sound one. A parent will be well rewarded for all the trouble if the limb remain only a little weak, instead of hanging as a useless flail, utterly incapable of doing any work at all.

In neglected cases the muscles contract, so that the leaders may require dividing, and the limb to be put into a surgical boot.

The paralysis itself never tends to get worse.

RHEUMATISM.

This disease is very apt to be overlooked, especially in young children, as the joint pains are often very slight, and are put down by the mother or nurse to " growing pains." The serious thing about rheumatism in young children is, that the heart is so very liable to become affected. Heart disease in children is always dangerous, and often fatal. St. Vitus' dance may follow an attack of rheumatism.

If a child complains of pains in its ankles, knees, or wrists, the best thing to do is to keep it warm in bed, and send for a doctor.

Inflammation of the covering of the heart is usually accompanied by vomiting, breathlessness, fever, and pain in the stomach.

CHAPTER XIII.

MEDICINES FOR BABY.

Medicines—Homœopathic Globules—Measure Glasses—Powders
—Aconite—Alcohol—Bicarbonate of Soda—Borax—Bromide
of Potassium—Calomel—Castor Oil—Chalk—Cod-liver Oil—
Dill Water — Glycerine — Ipecacuanha — Magnesia — Malt—
Manna—Opium—Parrish's Food—Rhubarb—Senna—Sulphur
—Compresses—Embrocations—Ointments—Poultices.

THE less medicine baby takes, the better will it be.
Baby's stomach was made for food, not medicines.
Many mothers seem to forget this, and are perpetually
dosing their unfortunate children with aconite, teething
powders, castor oil, etc. It is hardly to be wondered at
that such infants are never really well ; but it never
appears to dawn upon the mother that the remedies
employed are creating the very evils they are supposed
to avert.

All medicines should be kept in a place by themselves,
under lock and key, and every bottle properly labelled.
Nothing is safe from a child, and to have medicines,
liniments, and ointments lying about in the bedroom or
nursery is most dangerous, many a fatal accident having
occurred through want of a little forethought in this
matter.

Nurse should never be allowed to give any medicine
to baby, no matter how simple, without the knowledge
of the mother.

Medicines for children should always be given in as
palatable a form as possible. For this reason parvules,
tabloids, or granules (not homœopathic), are very convenient. The objection to giving homœopathic drugs is,
that one never knows what one is giving ; many of the
globules contain nothing but sugar, whilst others, though
really containing powerful drugs, do so in uncertain
quantities, and are therefore dangerous.

The usual mistake that a mother makes is this. Baby is ill; the disease is diagnosed (often wrongly), and baby is dosed with medicines that effected a cure in the case of some neighbour's or friend's child. Sometimes a medical or homœopathic dictionary is consulted, and the child is treated with all rigour according to the directions given.

In either case the child itself has been utterly ignored. The *disease* has been treated, and not the *child*. Children differ greatly in their constitution and requirements. Two children, both ill with bronchitis, may require exactly opposite treatment : the remedy that would save the one might kill the other. The great thing is to treat the *child*, not the *disease*.

Always carefully measure out the quantity of any medicine required in a proper medicine glass ; to guess haphazard is often dangerous, and to use ordinary spoons for measurement is always unsatisfactory. It is well to have two measure glasses, one a drop measure and the other for larger quantities.

The following table is approximately correct :—

60 drops equal one drachm, or teaspoonful.
120 drops equal two drachms, or one dessertspoonful.
4 drachms equal half-an-ounce, or one tablespoonful.
8 drachms equal one ounce, or two tablespoonfuls.
20 ounces equal one pint.

The best way to give a powder is to moisten the tip of one's finger, and when all the powder has adhered to it, introduce it into the child's mouth, as far back as possible. If a powder be at all nasty, mix it with a little finely powdered loaf sugar.

We will now look at a few remedies about which every mother ought to know something, in case of emergency, but it cannot be too much insisted upon that the only proper person to prescribe them is the doctor.

Aconite.—This is a most useful drug, and is often ordered in the treatment of the feverish attacks to which infants are so liable. When a child is feverish, with a hot, dry skin, and quick pulse, aconite will often act as a charm, quickly reducing the fever, slowing the pulse, causing perspiration, and enabling the child to get off into a comfortable sleep. It is, however, a depressing drug, and should not be given without medical advice.

Alcohol.—In the form of brandy, alcohol is an invaluable medicine for babies, though of course it should only be used on an emergency. To give wine, spirits, or beer to a child, as a regular thing, or because it seems to like them, ought to be rendered a criminal offence.

Brandy is most useful in cases of collapse, *e.g.*, after attacks of vomiting or diarrhœa. The dose for a child of one month old would be ten drops every four or six hours, diluted with three or four times the quantity of water. The quantity may be increased according to age, till at three months twenty to thirty drops every four hours for a few doses may be given just before food. Mixing it with a bottle of food is useless, firstly, because it is too much diluted to do any good, and secondly, because the child being ill, will probably only take a few mouthfuls, in which case it practically gets no brandy at all. Children respond to brandy in any form of prostration better than to any other stimulant ; it is also a useful sedative in the restlessness of teething.

Medicated wines, *e.g.*, coca wine or beef and iron wine, should never be given to children, and when in severe cases of illness brandy is being administered, it should always be called and treated as medicine.

Bicarbonate of Soda.—This remedy is chiefly of use in cases of acidity and flatulence. It is conveniently put up in tabloids containing five grains each. One of these dissolved in a teaspoonful of dill water and added to two teaspoonfuls of hot water, is a capital remedy for an attack of " wind " in a child of six months old. As before mentioned, bicarbonate of soda can be used for neutralizing acidity of milk, and a strong solution painted on a recent scald or burn quickly allays the pain. When a child's urine scalds and makes it uncomfortable, a dose of bicarbonate of soda three times a day will usually put all right.

Borax.—One ounce of borax dissolved in four ounces of glycerine makes an excellent application for painting the mouth in cases of thrush. Mixed with six times its volume of water, the glycerine and borax mixture makes an efficient gargle for older children.

Bromide of Potassium.—This is a nerve sedative, and is often of great service during teething.   It is also very useful for children who are excitable and nervous, and who talk and cry out in their sleep.   Bromide acts as a depressant on the system, and should never be given as a regular thing for any length of time.

Calomel.—This is a preparation of mercury which was at one time very largely used in the diseases of infants, but through misuse and abuse has fallen into undeserved disrepute.   If baby refuse its food, and the motions be clay-coloured, hard and dry, a dose of calomel at bed-time is often ordered, and will generally work wonders.

Cascara in the form of an elixir or syrup is a useful aperient in the chronic constipation of children, being given regularly for some time to act as an intestinal tonic.

Castor oil is one of the most efficient aperients for an infant : it has, however, the disadvantage of being somewhat constipating afterwards.   The dose for a child of six months old is half a teaspoonful.   A teaspoonful of olive oil is, however, in many instances, preferable to castor oil.

Chalk.—This drug is usually administered in the form of the aromatic powder, and is useful in cases of diarrhœa with acidity.

Cod-liver oil is a food rather than a medicine.   It may be employed in all wasting diseases, and given to children that are always having colds and coughs.   Thin, delicate children are often picked up and strengthened in a wonderfully short time by it.   An infant of a few months old can easily be made to take the oil by sucking at a finger which has been previously dipped in the medicine. To a child a year old a teaspoonful may be given twice a day after food.   It is a good plan to begin with a tea-spoonful, once a day, on going to bed.   With older children the dose may be increased to a dessertspoonful, which, if necessary, may be floated on milk, coffee, or orange wine.   It is of no advantage to give very big doses of the oil ; it will only repeat, and is not digested.

Kepler's extract of malt with cod-liver oil, and Scott's emulsion of cod-liver oil, are excellent preparations and easily digested.

Children with the least suspicion of rickets should take cod-liver oil all the year round, except in very hot weather. It is also a good preventive of chilblains in older children. Some children who will refuse cod-liver oil will take Virol, a preparation of bone marrow rich in animal fat.

Dill water.—Under this may also be considered, carraway, anise, and peppermint water, which are all good household remedies for the stomach-ache, colic, and flatulence. A teaspoonful, repeated occasionally if necessary, is the ordinary dose. An equal part of hot water added to the remedy, greatly enhances the effect.

Glycerine.—A teaspoonful in water at bed time often makes a good aperient for a child. Of late it has been the fashion to use an injection of this drug into the lower bowel, a special syringe being made for the purpose ; about a teaspoonful of glycerine is required, and it usually acts within five minutes. Suppositories containing glycerine are also employed, and are much less trouble. In quite young infants, the old remedy of introducing a small stick of soap into the anus is generally effective.

Ipecacuanha.—This drug is usually given in the form of the ipecacuanha wine. In large doses it acts as an emetic, that for a child of a year old being one tea-spoonful, repeated in fifteen minutes if necessary. In the treatment of croup it is often desirable to make a child vomit at once, and mothers, whose children are liable to that disease, had better keep a bottle of the wine in the house, so as to have it handy if required. It is often used in this way to clear the chest of phlegm in cases of bronchitis, or to empty the stomach in cases of over-feeding.

Ipecacuanha wine is not a drug that keeps well, and after some months is apt to make a deposit at the bottom of the bottle, and lose its good qualities.

Magnesia.—Probably the less aperient medicine a child takes, the more regularly will its bowels act. As pointed out elsewhere, the chief remedy for constipation is a change in the diet.

Magnesia, in the form of the citrate, or of Dinneford's fluid magnesia, is a harmless aperient if only used occasionally. In the summer weather, when a child gets easily upset, a dose of magnesia will often be very beneficial.

Malt.—There are several excellent preparations on the market, both with and without cod-liver oil, and children will readily take and digest them. They are especially indicated for thin children, with poor appetites and delicate digestions. Half a teaspoonful sucked from the finger or rubbed up with a little milk, will be greatly relished by an infant. For a child a year old a teaspoonful may be given twice a day.

Manna.—This is a very common household remedy for infantile constipation ; a teaspoonful dissolved in the bottle acts very well with some infants, but it is very uncertain, and with others will have no effect at all. A dessert-spoonful of prune juice is often efficacious with infants under a year old.

Opium.—This drug should never be given to children under any circumstances whatever, except by a doctor's order. Infants tolerate opium very badly, and thousands of young lives have been sacrificed to it, administered in the form of Soothing Powders, Composing Mixtures, Quieting Syrups, Paregorics, etc. No mother should be tempted ever to use any of these in order to keep her baby quiet ; they are poison, and should be avoided as such. A child who is always crying and sleepless cannot be well, and the mother had far better call in a doctor to point out what is wrong.

Two drops of laudanum have proved fatal to an infant, and a third of a grain of opium has killed a child of nine months.

Patent " soothing mixtures " are the cause of a great many of the inquests held upon children.

Parrish's Food.—This is a good pick-me-up for children over two years old ; it is best taken after dinner.

Rhubarb, though a very favourite household drug, is

not to be recommended for children, since when given as an aperient it proves constipating afterwards. It is usually given as a powder, or in the form of the syrup.

Senna.—Syrup of senna, though a good aperient, causes too much griping for infants of tender years.

Sulphur, in the form of flowers of sulphur, or the confection, is often of use to get a child's bowels into a proper condition. It should not be given under two years of age.

EXTERNAL REMEDIES.

It will be useful in conclusion to briefly consider a few of the external remedies which are commonly employed.

Compresses.—A compress consists of several folds of soft linen or calico wrung out of water, and covered with a piece of oiled silk or mackintosh sufficiently large to overlap the linen on all sides. Compresses are either hot or cold, according to the temperature of the water used.

In some cases, compresses have a sedative effect, calming a child's nerves and inducing sleep. One applied to the abdomen will often relieve constipation, and over the throat will usually relieve the aching of that part when sore.

Lotions.—Boracic lotion is a useful household remedy. It is good for bathing eyes which are inflamed from a cold, for cleansing little wounds such as those made by falling on gravel, and for applying on lint under oiled silk to gathered fingers. Evaporating lotion is made by mixing any spirit, *e.g.,* methylated spirit or Eau de Cologne, with four times its quantity of water. A single layer of linen or muslin can be dipped in this and laid on the forehead when a child is very feverish and restless, being changed as soon as it becomes dry. The same treatment is useful in the case of injury to a joint while waiting for the doctor.

Embrocations or *Liniments.*—In cases of cold on the chest, whooping cough, etc., it will often prove beneficial to rub the chest back and front, night and morning, with a simple liniment. An infant's skin is very easily irritated, so that no strong embrocation should be employed. Simple oil, camphorated oil, or a soap liniment diluted with oil, are about the best to use for this purpose. The rubbing should be performed with the child across the knees, in front of the fire.

Ointments.—Hazeline cream and Vinolia are perhaps the best ointments for nursery use in case of chafing, rough skin, or sores, but boracic or zinc ointments are also very useful.

Poultices.—These are much less used than formerly, but it is well to know how to make them properly. The material generally employed is freshly crushed linseed, or stale bread. The basin and knife should both be scalded in hot water, sufficient boiling water should then be put into the basin, and the meal gradually added, stirring all the time with the knife. The product should then be of the consistency of batter pudding, and be such that it can be easily spread on soft linen or old rag with the knife, to the thickness of about half an inch. The poultice should then be applied next the bare skin, and covered with one or more layers of thick flannel. A poultice thus made will keep hot for two or three hours, at the end of which time it should be removed, and, if necessary, a new one applied.

Of course a boiling-hot poultice should never be suddenly clapped on the tender skin of a child. Try the temperature of the poultice with the back of the hand, and then gently and gradually cover the required part.

Mustard may require to be added to the linseed; in which case it must be thoroughly mixed with the meal, or it will collect in one spot and produce a blister.

A poultice to cover the chest, which contains, say, a teaspoonful of mustard, should be partially removed after twenty minutes to see if the skin be sufficiently reddened. If so, remove it at once, or a large blister may occur before the danger is thought of.

After the removal of a poultice, the affected part should be covered with a layer of warmed cotton wool to prevent the child catching cold. On the chest the wool or poultice is best kept in place by means of a little flannel jersey.

A jacket poultice is one made to cover the entire chest,

back and front, coming well up beneath the armpits, and retained in place by a safety pin over each shoulder.

A good method of employing heat to relieve pain is to half fill an indiarubber hot water bottle with hot water, slip it into a flannel bag, and apply it to the painful part.

*   *   *   *   *   *   *   *

How to bring up a baby in a rational and scientific manner has now been briefly described, and in following the spirit rather than the letter of the foregoing pages, it is believed that mothers and nurses will prove the truth and wisdom of them in their own experience—*experientia multa docet.*

INDEX.

JOHN WRIGHT & CO., PRINTERS, BRISTOL.

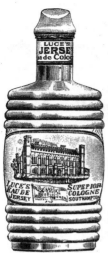

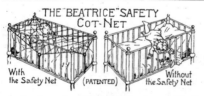

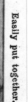

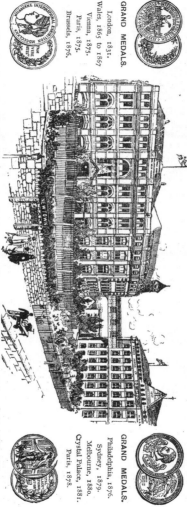

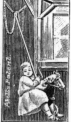

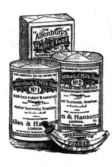

Ailments of Women and Girls.

◉◉◉

BY

FLORENCE STACPOOLE,

*Certificate Obstetrical Society, London; Lecturer for the National Health Society,
and for the Councils of Technical Education.*

NOTE.—The publishers have pleasure in stating that, as they anticipated, this little work has found many friends among those for whom it is written, and that the notices in the medical as well as the lay press confirm their own opinion that it is the simplest, safest and best book as yet issued in the English language upon the important subjects with which it deals, and that it can be recommended with the greatest confidence.

PRESS NOTICES.

"This book is an excellent example of its class . . . . . treats in a simple and straight-forward fashion of the various common ailments to which women are liable. There are many matters concerning their health upon which women are too often wofully ignorant, and many of their illnesses are brought on by neglect of the simplest precautions. Mothers are especially to blame in this respect and forget that their daughters require special supervision and instruction. The author is to be congratulated upon the clear manner in which she has described these various conditions, and upon the excellent common-sense of her recommendations. There are many hints in the book which will be of value to medical men, and it is one which we can cordially recommend to those for whom it is intended."—*Lancet.*

"There is a vast amount of good advice contained within the boards of Miss Stacpoole's book. No medical man will differ when she says 'an ounce of mother is worth a pound of doctor'—the sadness lies in the fact that so few mothers give their ounce of care to their daughters at the trying time of life."—*Scottish Med. Jour.*

"The knowledge it contains is calculated to save a great deal of suffering if properly realized. Especially in young girls, a good deal of suffering is caused by ignorance, and by a natural disinclination to explain their symptoms."—*The Queen.*

"Precision and clearness of expression, and a knowledge of the needs of those for whose instruction she writes. She has been exceptionally successful."—*Glasgow Herald.*

"As far as we can judge, nothing for the purpose could be better than this . . . . . a very useful book."—*News.*

"Well informed and clearly expounded in simple language . . . . . . cannot but prove helpful and instructive to women."—*Scotsman.*

BRISTOL: JOHN WRIGHT & CO.
LONDON: SIMPKIN, MARSHALL, HAMILTON, KENT & CO., LIMITED.

Fretful Babies.

Scores upon scores of young mothers are distressed and perplexed at the reason of a child's fretfulness. The mother thinks it is craving for food, and gives it in abundance, yet the fretfulness does not abate, and the child remains flabby, pallid, feeble, and puny, where it should be rosy, firm and growing. The secret is here. It is craving for food, but food of the proper sort. A child wants food containing a certain number of life-sustaining things, and if any one of those things is absent the child suffers. When proper food is given, a child is rarely restless, because it feels satisfied. Digestion is easy and natural, nutriment is rapidly absorbed, every part of the body is soothed, and healthy development takes place.

MELLIN'S FOOD

contains the proper proportion of everything necessary to infantile health and development.

"THE MOST PERFECT FORM OF COCOA."
—*Guy's Hospital Gazette.*

FRY'S

PURE
CONCENTRATED

300 Gold Medals, &c.

COCOA

Ask for the
" FIVE BOYS " MILK CHOCOLATE.

"Unrivalled as a Chocolate Confection."
—*Medical Magazine.*

Benger's Food

For INFANTS, INVALIDS, and THE AGED.

BENGER'S FOOD is quite distinct from any other obtainable. It is mixed with fresh new milk when used, is dainty and delicious, highly nutritive, and most easily digested. Infants thrive on it, and delicate and aged persons enjoy it.

The *Lancet* describes it as " Mr. Benger's admirable preparation."

The *British Medical Journal* says: " Benger's Food has by its excellence established a reputation of its own."

The *Illustrated Medical News* says: "Infants do remarkably well on it. There is certainly a great future before it."

From an Eminent Surgeon :—"After a lengthened experience of Foods, both at home and in India, I consider Benger's Food incomparably superior to any I have ever prescribed."

BENGER'S FOOD is sold in Tins by Chemists, etc., everywhere.

C

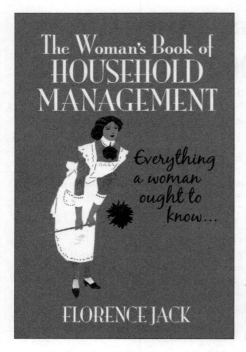

The Woman's Book of
Household
Management
Florence Jack

In the dim and distant past, when a Lady had servants to look after her house and there were no Kim and Aggie, she relied on the Edwardian bible for the household; the *Woman's Book*, a weighty tome full of useful information, hints and tips on how to run her household.

With everything from the price of setting up and furnishing a new home to how to clean, deal with the paperwork, remove stains, wash and iron clothes properly, and generally run a house in the Edwardian period, this book written in the rather formal style of 1911 is a mine of useful information, much of it still valid today.

978 0 7524 4210 5   £7.99

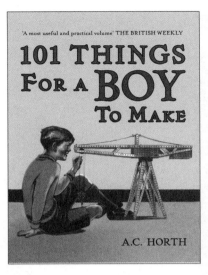

'A most useful and practical volume' THE BRITISH WEEKLY

101 THINGS FOR A BOY TO MAKE

A.C. HORTH

101 Things
For a Boy to Make
A.C. Horth

There are few boys who do not wish to make things, or who would not like to do some of the odd jobs to be found in every household, and it is for those boys who are on the lookout for suitable occupation that this book has been compiled. Whether it be a Spring-Operated Toy Machine Gun or a Garden Swing, this invaluable book originally published in 1928 captures the fascination and continual pleasure of making things for the active boy.

978 0 7524 4261 7 £9.99

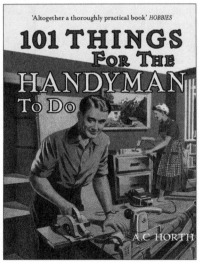

'Altogether a thoroughly practical book' HOBBIES

101 THINGS FOR THE HANDYMAN TO DO

A.C HORTH

101 Things
For the Handyman to Do
A.C. Horth

This volume caters for the man who likes to do odd jobs about the house and to spend interesting hours in making useful articles of furniture. Whether it be laying linoleum, making a concrete garden seat or re-stringing a racket, this invaluable book originally published in 1937 provides a wealth of helpful information for carrying out everyday repairs.

978 0 7524 4263 1 £9.99

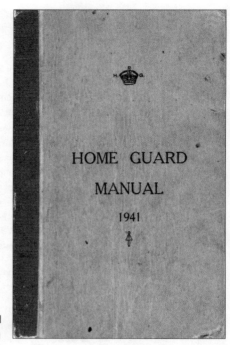

Home Guard Manual
1941

During the Second World War there was a call to arms that saw the founding of the Home Guard, a motley collection of men, poorly armed, many too old to fight. The Home Guard was untried in war, often without weapons or training, and they were Britain's last ditch defence against the Germans. But all was not lost and, over the period of a few months, this rag-tag group was armed, uniformed and trained using the *Home Guard Manual*. Taught basic fieldcraft, how to survive in the open, how to destroy tanks, ambush the invaders, use weapons of varying sorts, make boobytraps, read maps and send signals, the fledgling volunteer was turned into a veritable fighting machine.

978 0 7524 3887 0

£7.99